DANCING WITH THE BEAR

AND THE OTHER FACTS OF LIFE

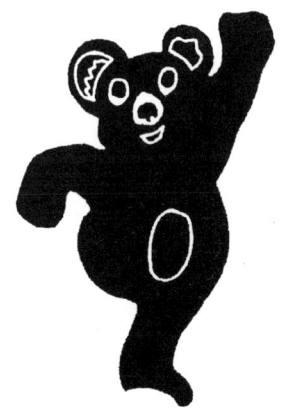

THE STORY OF
DR. M. JOYCELYN ELDERS
FORMER U.S. SURGEON GENERAL

BY HER BROTHER
CHESTER R. JONES

Copyright 1995 by Chester R. Jones
Pine Bluff, Arkansas
Published by Delta Press
416 National Building
Pine Bluff, AR 71601

All rights reserved. No part of this work may be reproduced in any form or by any means, except as may be expressly permitted in writing from Chester R. Jones

Printed in the United States of America

First Edition, 1995

Library of Congress Catalog Card Number: 95-074838

TABLE OF CONTENTS

ACKNOWLEDGMENTS..i
FOREWORD...ii
INTRODUCTION..1

PART I: THE EARLY YEARS

Chapter 1 Lil' Minnie's Birth: When and Where..............12
Chapter 2 Precious Mem'ries...21
Chapter 3 From the Hog Pen to the Washpot..................35
Chapter 4 Winter Sunset..48

PART II: HER GOLDEN PILGRIMAGE

Chapter 5 The First Leg of a Long Journey....................57
Chapter 6 Heroes 61
Chapter 7 Patriot..66
Chapter 8 Her Life's Vocation..69
Chapter 9 Work Ethic and Role Model............................73
Chapter 10 Anchored By Faith...79

PART III A WORK OF NOBLE NOTE

Chapter 11 Wind Beneath Her Wings..............................99
Chapter 12 A Call from the Governor.............................103

PART IV: UNLIKELY SUMMIT: U.S. SURGEON GENERAL

Chapter 13 A Call from the President............................109
Chapter 14 The Confirmation..112
Chapter 15 Short-lived Summit --No Place to Rest........166
Chapter 16 The Politics of Drugs, Race and Sex............177
Chapter 17 The Paradigm of Sex, Race & Sacrifice.........200
Chapter 18 Liberty Denied!...210

CONCLUSION: CONVICTIONS.......................................225
Works Cited 229

*Dedicated to our parents and first teachers,
Curtis and Haller Jones who taught us:
Joycelyn, Katie, Charles, Bernard, Chester, Beryl,
Pat and Phil,
living family values at home based upon
God's word in the Ten Commandments.*

and

*To the Methodist Women then,
now United Methodist Women,
whose support enabled my sister to develop the
philosophy:
Work like you don't need the money,
Love like there's no tomorrow,
Dance like nobody is watching.*

ACKNOWLEDGMENTS

I want to express my appreciation to my wife, attorney Valarie A. Jones, Associate Vice-President for Student Affairs at Virginia State College in Petersburg, Virginia; Bishop Richard B. Wilke and his wife, Julia, of the Arkansas Area of the United Methodist Church. I will never be able to repay Mrs. Wilke for continually encouraging her husband, my Bishop, until he made me a District Superintendent, the first African American in the 142 year history of the Little Rock Annual Conference. I have often said that if we had more women like Mrs. Wilke to encourage their husbands to be fair, we would not need an affirmative action program.

A special word of thanks is due to my nephews, Eric and Kevin, for their faithful and loyal support in helping and sharing with their Uncle Chess in the writing of this book. They both allowed me to interview them many times about growing up as the sons of Coach O.B. and Dr. Elders. Kevin, who was turned down on the appeal of his drug conviction by the Arkansas Supreme Court, will probably be in prison by the time this book is published. We should be thankful for Nelson Mandela who has taught us all that going to prison is not the end of the world.

I wish to extend my special thanks to President Clinton, whom I first met in 1978 when my brother, Dr. Bernard Jones, was kidnapped and killed in Little Rock. Then-Governor Clinton came and expressed words of condolence at the funeral and made a lasting impression on me and our whole family. I am grateful to the President for nominating my sister to be United States Surgeon General. My thanks go, also, to Senator Edward M. Kennedy who was very helpful in leading Dr. Elders through the Confirmation process. I, also, gratefully acknowledge the work of the millions of people who prayed, wrote letters of support and called their Senators in support of my sister's Confirmation.

I am especially indebted to Gina Teel, who God allowed to pass my way at the right time. She took a manuscript that I spent three years writing and made it come alive in three months. Gina is a very gifted editor, who I hope will still be available to assist me in completing my next book which should be out in early 1996.

Also I want to thank my "walking buddy" for six years, and great friend, Dr. Charles Donaldson, Vice Chancellor of the University of Arkansas at Little Rock. Dr. Donaldson is one of the most gifted persons that I know and should be the president of the largest corporation in America, yet he is totally committed to educating and teaching young college students in Arkansas. I am especially thankful for his vision in planning and helping to design the cover for this book.

My thanks to Dave & Ernie Wallis of Wallis & Wallis, Advertising, Pine Bluff, for the technical assistance in the printing of this book.

Last, but certainly not least, my very special thanks go to my Mother and Father, who gave all their children, "the courage to be."

Rev. Chester R. Jones

FOREWORD

M. Joycelyn Elders, M.D., a distinguished medical professional, thought-provoker and self-styled "lightning rod" intends to inspire protection of the public against those very difficult public health problems which threaten our well-being. She is a rare human being, a harbinger of change, a visionary who champions her cause.

We have worked together in Arkansas to lower tobacco sales, campaigning for higher tobacco taxes, because over 400,000 Americans die annually from tobacco related diseases. Against powerful lobbies, she courageously mobilized religious leaders and health care providers in this fight.

Her health concerns are rooted in her deep religious commitments. Her Methodist heritage and personal loyalty makes her angry when children aren't immunized, when children give birth to children, when "crack" or alcohol addicted babies fail to thrive. The vision of Jesus taking children in His arms makes her want to take all children in her arms and make them healthy and whole. The Methodist Social Creeds guide her social policies. She is an outstanding United Methodist.

There are those who may see her as crusader, missionary, modern-day prophet, advocate, or as a thorn in the side. No matter how she might be viewed, it is a fact that one commonsense theme permeates her discourse: preventive medicine and comprehensive health education. She states it this way, *"The emphasis in medical care and delivery must shift to the preventive mode in order to change the attitude of people toward their own personal health care."*

Her philosophies provide for a new beginning, a shift in the health care paradigm. The shift would mean a radical change in the way some people view health care and health care education. Change can be uncomfortable, but is not always bad. What she advocates offers more than just radical change; it offers hope.

As one of the nation's top health care professionals, Joycelyn Elders is eminently qualified to help mold the nation's health care policies and programs. She served the State of Arkansas as a faculty member at the University of Arkansas Medical Sciences (UAMS) College of Medicine and as director of the Arkansas Department of Health. Ultimately, she served her country as United States Surgeon General. She entered the University of Arkansas College of Medicine (now the UAMS College of Medicine) in 1956, and, with the exception of a one year internship at the University of Minnesota, received all her training in pediatrics at UAMS and Arkansas Children's Hospital. Before becoming Surgeon General, she developed a nationally recognized research and clinical program in endocrinology. She made seminal contributions in both basic and clinical research in diabetes and metabolic disease and was recognized by membership on national advisory committees, professional societies and study groups of the National Institutes of Health.

She worked to make the Arkansas Health Department into an active health service program by stimulating the formation of school-based clinics, community centers, etc. Of utmost importance, she dared—in a manner unlike anyone else—to address the major issues of teenage pregnancy, childhood immunization, AIDS, maternal/newborn care, access to care for the poor, teen violence, illegal drug use, etc. In all cases, she has opened the door for further debate of all the vitally necessary subjects.

While we may not agree totally with all Dr. Elders offers, she has seized whatever opportunities she could to prod us into addressing the very complicated social/health issues which we need to address. Though her race and sex might be considered handicaps by some people, Dr. Elders does not allow these factors to deter her. She was not afraid to use the "bully pulpit" of the Surgeon General's office to badger us into addressing the complexities of the social/health problems we face.

Does Joycelyn Elders know of what she speaks? You bet! She has seen it all. She grew up in economic poverty. There was no silver spoon for her. She knows what poverty without intervention can do to good people who are otherwise sound except for their inability to escape poverty. She assumed the office of Surgeon General coming from the small and poor state of Arkansas, which ranks near the top in the incidence of teen pregnancy; she personally has experienced the pain and knows as a mother what it is like to have the evil of illegal drugs infiltrate one's family. Joycelyn Elders knows of the social/health problems for which we are pressed to find solutions.

If history someday records M. Joycelyn Elders, M.D. among the country's most resourceful persons during the Twentieth Century, that assessment will be correct. She is highly knowledgeable, skilled, committed and uncompromising in her work. She is a realist when it comes to what she advocates. She is bold in her attempts to incite reform of health care thinking and the health care system in the country. In her powerful public speeches, she has forced us to open up discussion of once taboo subjects. This book will help readers know the person behind the presentations. It will help you know the forces that shaped her into one of America's leading physicians. She has enormous potential to be a major agent of change in health care for this decade and decades to come.

Today as we live and work in a world where our

children are going to hell on a bob-sled, while we hide behind stained-glass windows, untouched by the violence, Dr. Elders is out in the trenches fighting for the future of our children. I believe in the work Dr. Elders is doing. I believe she is a "voice crying in the wilderness," calling us all to task for our future and, especially, for the future of our children. I trust that this book will help us all to seriously consider her message, one that is vital for our future.

Bishop Richard B. Wilke
Arkansas Area
The United Methodist Church

INTRODUCTION

The Dance

Dancing with the Bear is an appropriate title for this chronicle of the life of M. Joycelyn Elders, M.D., former United States Surgeon General. It takes fortitude to outdance a bear. Dr. Elders certainly has fortitude!

As a pastor, many years ago, I heard the following old saying from a Methodist leader in Arkansas, Bishop Kenneth Hicks:

When you are dancing with a bear,
You can't get tired and sit down;
You must wait until the bear gets tired,
Then you sit down.

The wisdom of Bishop Hicks' saying really didn't register with me until recent years as I watched my big sister, Joycelyn, progress through her career and begin her dance with "the bear." You see, "the bear" is anything that seems insurmountable.

Who is M. Joycelyn Elders, M.D.?

Dr. Joycelyn Elders is the first African American and second woman to hold the highest medical post in the United States of America: U.S. Surgeon General.

The family tree of Dr. Elders shows that she is the firstborn of sharecroppers, the granddaughter of farmers, the great-granddaughter of slaves. It is said that our grandfather himself had to slip out of Louisiana into Arkansas. He worked on a farm and met and eventually married our grandmother. He and his bride moved to Howard County, Arkansas, near a little town called Schaal. Their eldest son (our father) was born shortly thereafter. Thus our family came to live in rural, Southwest Arkansas. Our parents remain in Schaal today close to the place where our grandfather came fleeing the aftermath of the Civil War and slavery in Louisiana.

Our family heritage, as that of most blacks in the United States, has its roots in slavery and has been forged in the decades since in trying to make our way in the world. Our family taught us the meaning and value of freedom, while still struggling against the many forces which infringed on our freedom because we were black, poor and living in the rural South. Our family lived the kind of life that many poor, black, Southern sharecroppers lived. We are proud of the heritage which is ours, but we are also ever aware of the painful realities which are a part of our past. There were times when it seemed we would not make it, but we learned to persevere. There is much about our life and our heritage that is hard to fathom from a late Twentieth Century perspective.

For instance, it may seem unbelievable that the nation's first African-American Surgeon General could be delivered by a rural, unlicensed midwife. Believe it! It is the truth! "Mother Sabie" served as the community's midwife because there were no doctors, white or black, in the area. Not one of the Jones' children would be delivered by a medical doctor.

On Sunday, August 13, 1933, Mother Sabie delivered Curtis and Haller Jones' first child. The baby, a six pound girl, was born in the heat of the summer in a house with no modern conveniences.

As a result of the poor conditions and the difficult birth, our mother had a hard time. This delivery would prove to be the most difficult birth of all her eight children. The baby girl was given the name Minnie Lee Jones (a name she would live with until her freshman year of college, when she legally changed her name to Minnie Joycelyn Jones). She would be nicknamed "Little Minnie."

Joycelyn Elders was born a daring and independent being. She dared to be born into this world under the watchful eyes of Mother Sabie, and she snapped triumphantly the chains of poverty when she graduated from the, then segregated and unequal, public schools of Howard County, Arkansas and left the farm armed with nothing more than faith, hope, a bus ticket and an address for Philander Smith College in Little Rock.

While at Philander Smith, she worked as a housekeeper to pay her room and board. A biology major, she set her sights on being a medical technician. It wasn't until she heard a speech by a young medical student that she even considered the possibility of becoming a medical doctor. That young student, Edith Irby Jones was the first black woman student at the University of Arkansas Medical School. After the speech, Joycelyn says she decided, "*I wanted to be just like her.*" Dr. Jones had become Joycelyn's first real role model, even though at the time Joycelyn may not have fully understood what the term meant. But now she realizes the importance a role model can make for young people and she takes her status as a role model very seriously.

Following her graduation from Philander Smith with a Bachelor of Science degree, Joycelyn Jones enlisted in the United States Army. She served as a physical therapist. After her honorable discharge, she later entered the Arkansas College of Medicine (now the University of Arkansas for Medical Sciences UAMS College of Medicine) on a G.I. Bill in 1956. She spent one year of internship at the University of Minnesota and returned to teach at

UAMS, where she has been ever since.

In 1987, then-Governor Bill Clinton asked Dr. Elders to be the Director of the Arkansas Department of Health. In the words of Harry P. Ward, Chancellor of the UAMS College of Medicine, *she remolded the health department into an active health-service program by stimulating the formation of school-based clinics, community centers, etc. Of most importance, she addressed the major issues of teenage pregnancy, childhood immunization, AIDS, maternal-newborn care, access to care for the poor, teen violence, etc. In many cases, her positions and opinions caused controversy. In all cases, she opened the window. At least we have been debating the right subjects.*
(UAMS Journal 2)

The Woman

As a young boy in Howard County, I developed a fondness and deep respect for my big sister. I thought she could do anything. I looked up to her. (I still do; she is *my* role model.) Yet there was always something about her. It wasn't that she wasn't warm, kind or caring when we were growing up, because she was all of these and more, but she was — well, she was just always different from everybody else. Back then I didn't know enough to try and figure her out as a person. I am not sure that I know enough today. But having shared so much with her over the last fifty years or so, I have had the unique opportunity to know her as a brother, friend, parishioner, confidant and supporter.

Whatever it was that fascinated me about my sister as a youngster fascinates me today. The difference is that I am now able to verbalize my views of what makes her so dynamic and distinctive to many, and at the same time so troubling to others.

Dr. Elders has always been imaginative; she is a woman

churning with ideas, and in a way her ideas have been radical. You could even call her a maverick. For example, she left the farm with virtually nothing, seeking a college education. Then she enlisted in the Army when it was almost unheard of for women—especially black women—to do so.

But my favorite example of her radicalism involves the time around 1957 when she was home visiting. She had taken our two younger sisters and me to see the movie "*Old Yeller*" at the local drive-in theater. When we drove up, Joycelyn refused to park in the back of the lot—in the "colored section." Instead, she parked on the edge of the white area. That was the first time I questioned whether she was a sane person. I thought she had gone to school and lost her mind. This was a time when Southern black folk had to know their place, stay in it, and not rock the boat. After we begged her and cried in fear, she eventually moved a space or two back into the "colored section" and grudgingly stayed for the movie.

That incident is a typical example of Joycelyn Jones then, and Joycelyn Elders today. She has always stood for what she felt was right for all people. Although she has had "a long row to hoe," she has been able to maintain the healthy blend of intelligence, energy, drive, boldness, strength, diligence, self-confidence, fortitude, independence, creativity, courage, and the solid work ethic necessary to propel her successfully through life.

While my sister is more a no-nonsense personality than not, she can be lighthearted. She has times when she likes to joke; she exudes warmth, is very kind, loving, thoughtful, and hospitable. You cannot find a better hostess. She is also dominant but not domineering. On the other hand, she is very rigid, disciplined and painstaking in whatever she does.

What she cares most about is people. She has a great desire to serve children. She believes every child should be a planned and wanted child. In her own words,

"If a child is a planned, wanted child, parents are going to do the best they can to make sure that child grows up healthy, educated, motivated with hope. If they don't want the child or didn't plan the child, then I think you have a far greater possibility that they will not be nurturing parents."

People have often asked me how Dr. Elders herself manages to be the loving and devoted wife and mother that she is, and at the same time be so involved in so demanding a career as hers. I usually respond, "she has a bucket full of energy."

In 1960, after a two month romance, she and Oliver B. Elders, then a basketball coach at a Little Rock high school, were married on Valentine's Day. They have two adult sons, Eric, a biology teacher in Pine Bluff, Arkansas, and Kevin, who lives in a half-way house in Fort Smith, Arkansas while awaiting the judicial process to be completed so that he can finish paying his debt to society.

Dr. Elders' life has been filled not only with triumph, but also with tragedy. Our brother, Bernard Jones, Arkansas' first black veterinarian, was murdered in 1979. Our sister Pat, a linguistics professor at Howard University, died in a car accident in 1986 while on assignment for the National Geographic Society on Johns Island, South Carolina. And Nina, a troubled young woman the Elders adopted at age 13, was found shot to death in 1993. Then, in 1994, came the arrest of her 28-year-old son Kevin on charges that he sold an eighth of an ounce of cocaine to an undercover police officer in Little Rock. He was found guilty of the charge in a non-jury trial. The conviction was appealed and was left standing by the state Supreme Court.

At this writing the judicial process continues. Through it all, Joycelyn has remained the family's rock. She knows what it is like to be wounded, but her faith in Almighty God allows her to keep on going.

Something else that I have observed about Joycelyn is her natural way with words. It is an art for her. She is outspoken, passionate and hard-hitting, but she is dedicated to the issues that are important to her. Her words have rankled established politicians and religious leaders, and have given T.V. commentators something to discuss on prime time and newspapers something refreshing to print. This quality has made her "public enemy number one" with some, especially with the so-called "religious right." The truth is that as a professional she is simply pragmatic about reproductive rights, care of children, public health care and education. Her words have simply infuriated those on the other side of the debate.

Dr. Elders has been called an "anti-Christian bigot," a "radical" (in the negative sense), a "way-out leftist," and "the condom queen" by certain groups. In fact, she is a medical doctor who happens to be African-American and who has a very strong and controversial resolve concerning the issues of teen pregnancy, AIDS, drug abuse, reproductive rights, and other health-related issues. It is unfortunate that such false perceptions still cloud our vision and breed sexism and racism, to which Dr. Elders is certainly no stranger.

It is ironic that some of those who so vehemently oppose some of her views would see fit to characterize her as an "anti-Christian bigot." To the contrary, it is her unshakable belief in God—along with a supportive husband—that sustains her through the various personal attacks she faces. Furthermore, she is an active member of the United Methodist Church, and she often echoes many of the

Church's positions in her messages. She received the support of several religious leaders during her confirmation hearing. Dr. Elders is a dedicated and practicing Christian. How can she be an "anti-Christian bigot" at the same time?

This is the Joycelyn Elders that I know!

The Content and Scope of the Book

"We see our children out in the ocean surrounded by the sharks of drugs, alcohol, homicide and suicide. We sit on the beach moralizing and talking about whose values should be taught, while our children drown . . . We have not addressed the needs and issues using up our children." This famous quotation from Dr. Elders' March 26, 1993 address to the Global Gathering, sponsored by the Board of Global Ministries of the United Methodist Church in Indianapolis, Indiana, gives a hint of the kind of hard-hitting message that has forced her into a "dance with the bear."

There are those who might characterize the former Surgeon General's work as a crusade, mission, campaign, prophecy, advocacy, etc. She calls it a responsibility. No matter how we may view her work, one common theme seems central to whatever her discourse: our emphasis in medical care must shift to the preventive mode in order to change the attitude of people toward their own personal health care.

Dancing with the Bear is a closer look at some of Dr. Elders' controversial positions concerning the very complex and troubling social/health problems that so many of us just do not seem ready to deal with. She has taken on the heavy responsibility of serving as a "lightning rod" to help protect all people from the troubling problems of teenage pregnancy, AIDS, teen violence, and other health crises.

She advocates policies, practices and programs which will improve health, educate people concerning their health, reduce risky behaviors and enable children to become healthy, educated, motivated and productive human beings.

Unfortunately, there are those who disagree with her, including influential religious groups, established politicians, and other conservative groups and individuals. These are "the bear" with which she must dance in order to get her message across. It has been a long dance for her; she is bloodied, but not bowed.

Joycelyn Elders believes she is somehow anointed to do what she must to help diminish the destructive effects of healthlessness, homelessness, huglessness, hopelessness and hunger. Far too many of America's inhabitants (including innocent children) have become members of what Dr. Elders has dubbed "The 5-H Club." She sees immeasurable opportunity for Americans to gain control of their lives and radically alter the effects of the 5-H Club. But, she says, *"we have got to do more than offer rhetoric."*

If history is fair to Dr. Elders, there is at least one accomplishment that it has to record in her favor. She was able to open the way for bringing the hard reality of very sensitive social/health problems and issues out of the closet and into the open.

Dancing with the Bear is about Dr. Elders' plan for improving the quality of health care in the country. At the heart of this book is a caring crusader's cry for change: change in the way we view and deliver health care in America. Whenever she speaks, if we can dull our taste for racism, sexism, and all of the other "isms," we can hear her assurance that *"we can change if we choose to change."*

Whether the philosophies, programs and policies that Dr. Elders advocates are useful in improving public health in America depends largely upon whether parents, school officials, government leaders, religious leaders, and the public in general are also willing to "dance with the bear" instead of "putting on Band Aids when we need major surgery." Dr. Elders readily admits that bringing her vision to reality requires coalition-building and that she spends a great deal of her time recruiting the support of churches, schools, civic organizations, judges, businesses, local communities, states, any and everyone she can get to join the dance. Her philosophy provides for a new beginning and a shift in the health care paradigm. The shift necessitates a radical change in the way we view health care. It is certainly clear to those who care to see that the present way is not working. In her message, Dr. Elders offers more than just a radical approach to change; she offers hope. It is something we have seldom seen before. What she proposes requires people to change their lifestyles. It requires us to perform major surgery on our attitudes concerning health care.

To demonstrate her point, she has stated that it is foolish to continue to spend approximately $900 billion a year on health care, but less than 1% of it on preventive health care. Further, she adds, "*90% of this $900 billion is spent on care during the last month of life. So we aren't paying for health, we are paying for dying.*"

Dancing with the Bear provides an authentic look at Joycelyn Elders' life, her statements and her ideas about how to reform concerns regarding social/health problems into *commitment* to do something about the situation. It seeks to provide a closer look into Joycelyn Elders the person, the doctor, the former Surgeon General, where she came from and where she is headed. Reading *Dancing with the Bear And The Other Facts of Life* will afford readers the chance to

- learn for themselves who Joycelyn Elders is and what she is really about;
- know more about the challenges that the nation faces in the area of health care as we enter the 21st century;
- improve perspectives on individual and collective responsibility for the protection of self and others through preventive health care;
- understand how "dancing with the bear" is really a process of change; and
- understand why improving the quality of health care can no longer be left to ignorance.

It is a health care thing! *Dancing with the Bear* brings the point home. It is past time for us to take off the blinders and deal with the issue. America has a health care crisis on its hands. Expanded vision and more progressive thinking are musts as we face the new century. The general public must mobilize and be willing to cut in and "dance with the bear." Will you dance?

While we ponder, M. Joycelyn Elders, M.D., can't get tired; she can't sit down. "The bear" is not tired yet!

Rev. Chester R. Jones

Chapter One

LI'L MINNIE'S BIRTH: WHEN AND WHERE

It's up to each man what becomes of him,
He must find in himself the grit and vim
That brings success; he can get the skill,
If he brings to the task a steadfast will...
(Anonymous)

Forged in Steel

My mother once said she believes the hard times back on the farm may have steeled her eight children, and no one is tougher than her eldest child. For a long time, I struggled to understand what she really meant by that statement. It puzzled me so much that I asked her once what she meant. She meant that the hard times had created in her children a strong resolve, or determination, to outfox poverty itself by leaving the tenant-farm life, getting a good education, and striving to be somebody. Whew! What a relief! I guess I wanted reassurance that we're OK; that Momma thinks we're OK.

Momma's statement haunted me most when my big sister, M. Joycelyn Elders, M.D., came under such blistering fire for simply stating what she believed and taking firm positions on certain issues. It can be disquieting, to say the least, when you grow up believing literally in the American dream, the Constitution of the United States, the Bill of Rights and freedom of speech and later learn that what is written is not always meant for everyone—or at least the interpretation and application of the Constitution doesn't seem to be the same for everyone—particularly minorities and women. But Momma knew better than I; she understood that the world is not always fair and that it is our early learning and experiences which forge us into the sort of people who can meet with grace and dignity whatever adversity or success comes our way.

Momma's statement still causes me to be curious about how my big sister remembers life on the farm. Does she remember it as a forging ground for the nerves and will of steel which she must have to survive in today's tough world? So, when time permits, I will engage her in conversation about the way things were when we were growing up. She doesn't always seem as emotionally involved in the subject as I am. In fact, she seems rather dispassionate when she talks about our childhood. The memories are sometimes painful, and perhaps we would all like to have a somewhat different past to remember. Also, perhaps, her reticence has to do with the fact that she never really had a childhood in the traditional sense, because, as a child, Joycelyn had to learn how to work before she ever learned how to play. Being the oldest of eight children, she was always either taking care of those of us who were younger, or working in the cotton fields. I think that she also realizes now, in talking about our childhood, how far our parents went to protect us from racism and discrimination. Joycelyn was never allowed, or perhaps never wanted, to get lost in a world of little girls' daydreams like most little girls do. She never dreamed of herself being the center of some Cinderella-like fairy tale. She knew that in order to succeed she would have to work hard. So, even though Joycelyn exhibits a degree of reticence, one quickly gets the feeling that she holds much pride and joy regarding our childhood. She will readily remind a listener that

"our parents taught us honesty, self-esteem, and integrity. It was a real strong virtue to work hard and to always do your best."

Our parents had instilled in us the knowledge that we

could do anything we wanted, if we were willing to pay the price for it.

These attitudes were ingrained in my sister and have seemed to stick in her mind like a mantra throughout her life. It is quite obvious that Joycelyn must have clearly understood at a very early age that it was up to her to determine what would become of her. That understanding might have seemed lofty for a sharecropper's daughter, but there can be no doubt that she possessed the "grit and vim" that lead to success. She was taught to believe that in every cloud there is a silver lining, and in every disadvantage there is an advantage.

Throughout Joycelyn's life, it has been evidenced that her steadfast will is a driving force in her. Today, considering all her accomplishments, who can justifiably doubt her skills? She earned the highest professional degree in her field—the Doctor of Medicine degree—and board certification to go with it. On the one hand, her success stands in contrast to her beginnings. On the other hand, I continue to believe that her life epitomizes the American dream, and more especially it proves our parents correct in what they taught us.

Humble Beginnings

Certainly Joycelyn came from the humblest of beginnings, but yet there is a real sense of pride which is a part of our family's heritage. Joycelyn is the firstborn of our parents, Curtis and Haller Jones, the paternal granddaughter of Charlie and Minnie Jones, and the maternal granddaughter of Charlie and Elnora Reed. Charlie Jones never talked much about his father, who was a slave in Louisiana. It is said that Charlie Jones himself was slipped out of Louisiana into Arkansas in a pine box. Once in the state, he made his way to Ozan, Arkansas, where he worked on a farm until he met his bride-to-be, Minnie. They married and moved to Howard County, Arkansas, near a little town called Schaal. Schaal (pronounced "shawl") is located in Southwest Arkansas, some twenty-four miles from Hope, the birthplace of President William Jefferson Clinton. The firstborn of Charlie and Minnie was a son whom they named Curtis.

Curtis and Haller met and fell in love as mere teenagers. The two were married on August 29, 1932. Given their limited education and the general life situation of Negroes at the time, it seemed they were already destined to be sharecroppers. Curtis and Haller Jones each completed only the eighth grade. Curtis' education was interrupted by his family's need for him to work. Like so many Negroes of the time, he gave up education for work in the fields, not by choice, but because the family's economic condition required it.

The newlyweds found a place to live on land they did not own. It was owned by the Hill brothers and called the Hill Brothers' Place. The house was a small one room shack with a tin roof. It was located between Mine Creek and the Saline River; it was also the home of the largest mosquitoes in the state of Arkansas. Curtis and Haller worked the land for a share of the crop (a small share). They had fallen in love, married and set up housekeeping during the worst of economic times, the Great Depression, and most Negro families in southern Howard County, as the old saying goes, "didn't have a pot to pee in." They were poor and worked other people's land. Those who understand what it meant to be a sharecropper know that the tenant-farmer, particularly in the South, was given credit by the white land and store owners for seed, tools, living quarters and food. They worked the land and received an agreed-upon share of the value of the crop, minus charges. It may be argued that this was just another style of Southern slavery, but it was what poor Negroes had as a means of employment. There are still sharecroppers in some places; but, back then it was an even more unfair system in terms of the compensation given for the output of the poor workers.

Our mother was often ill during the pregnancy with Minnie. "Mother Sabie" was the only health care provider we had at the time. She took care of Momma's medical needs as best she could. She served as the community's midwife because there were no black doctors in the area, and Negroes (the acceptable description of the race at the time) held a basic mistrust of Caucasian doctors. The fear was that they would sterilize the Negro women. Not one of the Joneses' children was delivered by a medical doctor.

It was slightly more than one year after her parents' teenage marriage that Li'l Minnie Jones was born in her maternal grandmother's house and bed. On Sunday, August 13, 1933, toward late evening, she was the first of eight children to be born to Curtis and Haller Jones, ages 18 and 15 respectively. Li'l Minnie made her way into this world almost before Mother Sabie could arrive to assist with her birth. When Haller's water broke, Curtis was told to run and get Mother Sabie. When Curtis returned, the baby, a six pound girl, was already well on her way. It was a hot summer day. The temperature had been in the 90's most of the day, and not a breeze could be felt anywhere. There was no fan, electricity or running water in the house.

For a while, Mother Sabie feared the baby might not survive the birth. Following the rough ordeal, it seemed a miracle that both mother and child did survive. As a result of the poor conditions and the difficult birth, Haller developed a fever and bled severely, but she pulled through it all by the grace of God and under the watchful eyes of Mother Sabie. This delivery would prove to be the most difficult birth of all her eight children. Momma would give birth to seven more children before she turned thirty. The baby girl was given the name Minnie Lee Jones, for her paternal grandmother (a name she would live with until her freshman year of college, when she legally changed her name to Minnie Joycelyn Jones). She was generally called "Li'l Minnie" by most adults.

There was no earthly way anyone who witnessed the birth of Li'l Minnie could have realized that the little sharecroppers' daughter would one day rise from the clutches of poverty surrounding her birth and become the first African-American to serve as the United States Surgeon General. The story of how Li'l Minnie escaped poverty and desperation to go on and become Surgeon General is the American story. It is the story of the house of her birth which lacked such comforts as electricity, indoor plumbing or natural or butane gas, but where there was plenty of pride and hope to enable a young girl to believe in her ability and her possibilities. It is the story of hard work and perseverance. It is not the trite story of many miles walked through feet of snow to get to school. It is the real story of how one, with enough drive and determination, can come up from the depths of poverty.

After a couple of months, our mother was finally able to make the trip from our grandfather and grandmother's house to the little shack on the Hill Brother's place. She rode on the back of a horse holding Li'l Minnie while my father walked in front leading the horse. Once they got settled back into their little house they quickly realized that they would need to make some special adaptations for a new baby. The mosquitoes were still bad, and their presence was intolerable with a new baby in the house. Our father had to go to Mineral Springs, some five miles away, to Dillard's Dry Good Store to buy material to make a mosquito net to cover up Li'l Minnie. The Dillard family who owned the dry goods store were Tom and Hattie

Dillard, parents of the present head of Dillard's Department Stores. Tom and Hattie Dillard were important people in Mineral Springs. Momma says that they were some of the best people in the world for giving credit to everyone in the community until harvest time. William Dillard and my father used to go swimming together down at the old swimming hole near the railroad trestle. The Dillards were real role models in relating to all people with dignity and a sense of human worth in the sight of God, regardless of color. We could all learn an important lesson in race relations from their example. They were people who dared to go beyond the bounds of expected behavior to be truly inclusive. I know that in recent times the Dillard Company has come under criticism around the area of race relations. What I have to say is that if this is a problem, which I have not personally experienced, I know that it is not a result of anything Mr. Dillard learned from his parents. People like the Dillards were a real help to my family in those early days. They helped to make life easier for young parents whose new responsibilities required a lot from them.

Charlie and Elnora Reed, the maternal grandparents of Li'l Minnie, had become very attached to their firstborn grandchild and did not want her to live in the small, one-room tenant shack. Elnora decided her granddaughter just could not live in the shack during the coming winter. She impressed upon Momma and Daddy that they needed to move into Uncle Jeff Reed's place. Uncle Jeff, like so many other Negroes in the area, had left Schaal during the depression and migrated to Chicago in search of a better life.

Uncle Jeff's little house was surrounded by forty acres of good timber and farmland and one of the best water wells in the area. The little place was located closer to good game areas, which would be useful for Daddy's hunting and trapping. Also, about three miles away, there was a store, a little post office and the church where Li'l Minnie would later attend school. Momma and Daddy were more than happy to move into Uncle Jeff's place, a three-room house. They considered it a real blessing to have their own little place, and not to be told by someone else what they could and could not plant.

The family later moved to the Will Jones place. By this time, our sister Katie was born, followed by Charles and Bernard, myself (Chester Ray), Beryl, Pat, and baby brother Phil. The same midwife, Mother Sabie, assisted with all the births.

Our sister Pat, I remember, had a chronic case of asthma as a child. She would cough and wheeze something awful sometimes. I can remember that my sister Minnie would help Momma burn some kind of green substance in a fruit jar lid when Pat would start coughing. The smoke from whatever the substance was seemed to help Pat breathe easier during these attacks. Minnie would fan the smoke up while Momma held Pat over the burning substance in order to get her to inhale. There were times when Pat's asthma was so bad that she would curl up in a ball like she was going to die. I think that her condition was complicated by the fact that she was exposed to the cold. Once, I know, she caught a bad case of pneumonia due to exposure to the cold. There was only one fireplace in the house, in Momma and Daddy's bedroom, and the cook stove in the kitchen. At night after the cooking was finished the one bedroom was the only warm place in the house. We would go in and get warm by the fire in the fireplace and wrap up in a blanket or quilt and run and jump in bed to try to stay warm. Often there were three or four of us in one bed which helped to stay a little warmer, but the constant exposure to the cold of an unheated, drafty room made Pat's problems worse.

Our family was fairly typical of most of the sharecroppers of that time. We did what we had to do to survive. We didn't have any luxuries—not even the luxury of a doctor when we were ill, unless it was a matter of life and death. We knew how to make the most of the little we had and we learned to work hard in order to have anything. But in spite of how little we had, our parents instilled in us the belief that we could have more if we worked for it. We may have lacked in material wealth, but we didn't lack for ambition. In fact, the sharecropper's lifestyle never seemed to diminish Daddy's ambition to own his own land; if anything, the poverty only seemed to increase his aspirations. Daddy was a proud, well-built man, as strong as a bull. He always seemed to take so much pride in paying his poll tax so he could vote. We were also proud for him.

Our experiences growing up gave us the tools we needed to do well in life. We were taught hard work, pride in our work, honesty, independence and ambition. These things would see us all through life in good stead. We learned these lessons from the earliest days of our lives. Minnie, being the firstborn, learned them very well and helped to teach the rest of us.

Chapter Two

PRECIOUS MEM'RIES

> *Universal, early childhood education will prepare our children to learn and achieve, removing some of the disadvantages that hold them back. At age four, a child knows half as much as he will ever know....*
>
> Dr. M. Joycelyn Elders
> ("Portrait" 8)

The Ritual of Hard Work

The early years of Little Minnie's life were spent in the simple but hard Southern sharecroppers' family lifestyle. As a young child, she had to work hard, and often keep pace with the grown folk. She shared in chores such as pulling corn, stripping cane, sawing wood with a crosscut saw, baling hay, milking cows, slopping hogs, pulling peanuts, digging potatoes, picking vegetables, plowing fields, canning foods, etc. She started picking cotton when she was only five years old, and had a quota of cotton to pick every day just like everybody else. It was not at all unusual for her to help daddy stretch coon hides and build fires in the fireplace or the wood-burning cook stove.

Things were done according to what seemed like rituals back then. For instance, we would get up early when the rooster crowed. Sometimes people would joke that when the hens had angered the old rooster before the chickens had gone to roost for the night in the tree above the hen house, the old rooster would make us all pay by crowing an hour or two earlier the next morning. True or not, the ritual was that when the rooster crowed, it was time to get up and start the day. Almost before the rooster had finished crowing, you could hear Daddy say, "Mint, get up!"

After hearing Daddy's call to Mint (another nickname for my oldest sister), I'd lie there for a few minutes listening to the music of the fireplace as the kindling wood blazed and the wood cinders crackled. When the fire had warmed the house, the younger ones would get up and dress around the fireplace and start to the barn to do their chores.

As for Mint, her day began with performing certain chores and then going to the pasture to catch the mules and harness them up and hook them to the wagon before breakfast. After breakfast she would go to the fields with Momma and Daddy and work until sundown. Part of the land farmed by the Joneses was located three miles from where we lived. Mosquitoes were plentiful. Snakes were everywhere, especially spreading adders, coach whip and cotton-mouth water moccasins. The spreading adder could make its head flatten out like a bedspread when it sensed trouble. The coach whip could stick its head above the grass and whisper when anyone got too close. These two snakes had a reputation for being bad, but only the cotton-mouth water moccasin posed a real threat. Also in the summer, ticks and chiggers were major culprits we had to contend with. I never figured out why God made chiggers until I went through the Confirmation process with my sister. My mother would take turpentine to the field with her to put on our insect bites.

Momma, Daddy and Minnie would ride to the fields in a horse-drawn wagon with iron wheels. The ride would usually take about 45 minutes down a gravel road, across the train tracks and through the woods. Once they were there they worked a hard day of plowing, planting, hoeing and picking, depending on the season.

At the end of the day, Momma and Minnie prepared supper. Since we had moved to the Will Jones' Place, Momma always had a big garden filled with a variety of vegetables. There were also home-cured meats, chicken, etc. Momma and Minnie canned a lot, so there were jars of peaches and all kinds of preserves for the hot hoecakes and biscuits. We never went hungry a single day in our lives.

After supper, the family would enjoy time together—usually fellowship and study—in our parents' room where the fireplace was. We were made to take warm baths and sometimes the babies would take a little nap before bedtime. Some evenings we enjoyed cornbread crumbled in buttermilk, or tea cakes and milk. On a cold night, we would all gather around the fireplace and bake sweet potatoes, parch peanuts, cook hominy grits and watch the fire burning in the fireplace. I remember that ash wood seemed to be the best for faster burning. Small pine kindling was used to start the fire and a big piece of oak, called a "backstick" was placed on the fireplace at night before going to bed to keep a slow fire going all night. Sometimes the fire would go completely out anyway. It was always the oldest child's job to start the fire in the morning, which meant that Minnie was responsible for getting the fire going every morning to cook and keep us warm.

Simple Play

Children growing up in Minnie's day had to be creative. For example, we were too poor for our parents to spend money buying commercially made toys. Our toys, rather, were custom-made. The older children made their own toys from wood and whatever else they could find in the junk piles. My brothers and I made spool toys from empty thread spools and rubber bands. Soapy water was used to lubricate the toys so we could engage in competitive matches. These kinds of things made life full of clean and wholesome fun. Children really enjoyed competing and playing with each other in those days. I remember one of the treats that our father would bring us back from town after selling a bale of cotton was a box of Cracker Jacks. This was a favorite snack for most children in the community. The box of caramel-covered popcorn was a great treat over regular popcorn because there was always a special surprise gift inside. Most of the gifts were only small, cheap plastic toys or cards. It was always like solving a mystery to sift through the box while eating the popcorn in order to find the anticipated gift. Whenever Minnie found the mystery prize she would always show it off to everyone around. The prize was always a valued treat, a great discovery. The box of Cracker Jacks, "junk food" by our standards today, was our favorite snack with its surprise gift, trinket, and it also provided us an outlet for expectancy while searching for the mystery of the prize. It seems today that most children have lost the expectancy, mystery and excitement that we had in our childhood. Most of the children in our cities today live dull and monotonous lives with little sense of expectation. Mystery and expectancy are vital parts of a child's life. The boxes of Cracker Jacks put enjoyment and expectancy into our lives.

Holidays and Hope

The other time of the year when there was a great sense of expectancy for us was at Christmas. The holidays would break the everyday routine and held the promise of something new and different. Christmas put life into our tired bodies. There are no words that can adequately capture the essence of what Christmas meant to us as children. It meant more to us than gifts and presents. It meant fun time with family around the fireplace, going to visit grandma and grandpa, decorating the tree, a big meal together, church.

I remember that the search for Christmas trees was a community event. I remember going out into the back woods with a group from the community looking for Christmas trees to cut down and bring home. We would find the perfect tree, saw it down and hurry home to put it up and decorate it. Then, I remember, on Christmas morning the excitement of seeing the presents underneath the tree. We would all gather around waiting in anticipation for the magic moment to arrive when the presents would be opened. Of course, we never knew what we would get for Christmas until Christmas morning after Santa Claus had made his rounds. We didn't make long lists for our parents like children do today, so we didn't know in advance what we would receive. For our parents, like other families at that time, what we would get depended on how the crops had done that year, how much game my father had trapped for the hides, etc. But there was always something for us under the tree on Christmas morning. Santa Claus always came after we were put to bed at night. One year, it must have been while Minnie was home from Philander Smith, I got up out of bed and sneaked back to the door to watch through the keyhole for Santa. My father must have seen or heard me, because he whispered to Minnie who got some ashes from the fireplace and crept up beside the door. She bent over and blew the ashes through the keyhole right into my eyes. I remember that Minnie would take us younger kids out and show us the tracks where Santa had ridden his sled clean up to the chimney. I still remember seeing the tracks made by Rudolph the Red Nosed Reindeer and the rest of Santa's team. I still don't know whether Minnie got up early and led our mules around in the yard intentionally to make those tracks, or what. At any rate, it was fun being a child at Christmas because we really believed that the mule tracks that Minnie showed us were the tracks of Santa's reindeer.

I remember the Christmas that I received my first bicycle. It was a second-hand bicycle that my Aunt Joe in Kansas City sent for me. I always had a special connection with that aunt after that Christmas. We would often get a new cap pistol or maybe a B-B gun. We always had fireworks at Christmas, that was the only time of year we had them then. We had apples and oranges and nuts, our favorite was brazil nuts that we called "n" toes. If there was snow we would have snow ice cream, a real treat.

Mostly, Christmas was a family time. We would get together and remember the baby born in Bethlehem. My grandmother would tell us the Christmas story. We would go to church and listen to the preacher talk about the baby Jesus and the star that marked the place he was born and guided the magi. We would go outside at night and pick out a particularly bright star in the sky that we were sure must have been the star of Bethlehem. We would have a big family feast as part of our celebration. We would have baked hen and dressing, a raccoon, if Daddy got one, with sweet potatoes (Momma would leave the raccoon's head on for our Christmas feast), coconut cake and sweet potato pie. Momma's recipe for raccoon was to skin the coon; take the musk ball out, if they were not taken out the varmint would be strong and taste too "coony"; soak over night in salt water to get all the blood out and leave the meat white; then put it in a pot with water, onion, salt and pepper and boil until tender; after this step the coon would be taken out and placed in a roasting pan and roasted in the oven sprinkled with black pepper and surrounded with sweet potatoes. I can still smell it all cooking and remember how good it all tasted to us because we had worked hard to get it.

Christmas was, for us, a time of hope. It gave our family an important sense of identity. There was a cohesiveness and stability that came out of that yearly celebration.

Christmas, more than any other season, seems to epitomize the excitement and wonder of childhood. I've always loved the Christmas season best because it meant so much to us as children. I guess the Christmas season still brings out more of the child in me than any other time. I think that we need that sense of excitement, wonder and hope. There weren't a lot of those extraordinary things around for us on a daily basis, I guess that's why Christmas meant so much. We could dream and feel excited and hopeful. Christmas really helped to set the tone for the next year.

After the excitement and hopefulness of Christmas the New Year would always challenge us to believe that life held some good things for us. We always looked forward to the coming of the new year. The scripture from the Book of Revelation, "Behold, I make all things new" (Revelation 21:5 KJV) was one that we could claim with hope. New Year's day always brought the special lucky treat meal of ham hocks and black-eyed peas. In actuality, this meal did little to help face the mountains of challenges and anticipated troubles, but we always looked forward to it and, for that one day, we seemed to have an extra measure of hope that things would become new and different.

Ways of Making an Honest Dollar

Besides what our family earned by sharecropping and working in the fields, we depended on trapping for an additional source of revenue. Minks, raccoons, opossums, fox and other fur-bearing animals were means of making money for us. My father would take me trapping with him. We would trudge through the woods to the traps he had set out in hidden places, sometimes baited to catch an opossum or fox. When we went from one trap to the next we had a sense of eager anticipation. The next trap must surely have something, and, of course, we always hoped especially hard that it would be a mink in the next trap.

Opossums were fairly easy to trap. They would almost always be caught in the trap by a front foot. The opossum would give up on trying to get away and be in the trap when we came. A raccoon, however, would not give up until it had gnawed its foot off to get out of the trap. It would go through desperate mutilation to gain freedom.

A good dog was also important to us in hunting and trapping animals. There were two things my father hated, a dog that would suck eggs and a hog that would eat chickens. Daddy felt that a dog that would suck eggs would not hunt and a hog that would eat chickens would eat young baby pigs. So he would kill them both. Daddy liked to keep a good coon dog. He had a bull horn he would blow and call his dogs when it was time to quit the hunt and go home.

One animal that we didn't want to meet up with in our hunting and trapping was a polecat, or skunk. An old polecat will spray you with the worst smell you ever smelled. They are the prettiest animals in the world, with that lovely black and white striped back, but watch them when they raise their tails. My friend Doyle Rogers, a successful businessman with the Wal-Mart Corporation, tells the story about when he was trading in furs. One day he and his wife, Raye, were driving home and he stopped the car to pick up a dead skunk on the road. He put the skunk in the back of the car and sold the hide for $2.00. "But," he said, "*I had to hold my nose every time I would ride in the car for the next two weeks.*" A pretty high personal price to pay to earn $2.00. Of course, when we were growing up that would have been a lot of money.

Different Kinds of Wealth

In those days there were no designer clothes, name brand sneakers or starter jackets for us. We wore many hand-medowns or second-hand clothes. The rest of the clothes we wore were handmade by the women in the family. At the beginning of the school year, each of us usually did receive a new pair of shoes.

We certainly didn't have anything that could be considered real luxuries until after Minnie had left home. One of the first real luxuries we had was an outhouse. An outhouse was not an affordable item and was considered a luxury by our father as long as we had woods within a mile of the house where we could go. We never had an outhouse at home until Minnie's last year of college and we moved to our Grandmother Minnie's home after our grandfather died. To have an outhouse was a status symbol, which meant the family who owned one had a lot of money. In the early forties and mid-fifties very few black families in rural Southwest Arkansas had an outhouse. I, even to this day, ask myself why? It is not that an outhouse was hard to build. It is one of the most basic facilities in life, yet this little chicken-coop-like facility, with a slanted roof, set down by the hog pen, was considered an impossible dream for most blacks in rural Southwest Arkansas at that time. It was something they would get when they arrived in the Promised Land, or in Heaven. And I am told that no one will need an outhouse, toilet, latrine, bathroom or "john" in Heaven. In Heaven you will only need the old Sears & Roebuck Catalog.

We may not have had a lot of toys, clothes and material things, but we had as much as the other people around us. Yet in spite of the fact that we were impoverished when it came to material things, we were rich with love, family time together and hard work to make our way in the world. Perhaps we would be better off today with a little less material riches and a little more of the kind we had when we were growing up.

Sex Education? Mostly Morals

So far, I have described many of the positive aspects of the early years of our family life. We come now to a point I know many have wondered about, since it relates to Dr. Elders' strong stand on certain sensitive sexual issues, and to her own upbringing, background and learning about these issues. The curiosity might be framed in a question like this: "I wonder what kind of parental guidance she received as a child?" Well, the truth is that when we were young children, parents didn't talk much about "the birds and the bees." Of course, when girls and boys became what parents considered "age appropriate," we were made to understand that if we did certain things, certain things would happen, and both the behavior and the results were totally unacceptable. Most of the sex education in our time was, in actuality, morality and value training. The issues around sex were seen mainly as moral, even theological, issues at that time. We didn't understand the need for education about the physical, medical, social aspects of sex and sexuality.

For the most part, children were taught that sex outside marriage was a sin. The general principle handed down from generation to generation was that one should wait and save oneself for marriage; if a couple were that much in love and simply couldn't wait, then perhaps it was time to request parental consent for an early marriage. It was a "no-no" and a sin to even think about sex and let it be known. Human sexuality being what it is, and the sex drive being what it is, children were often left with a sense of helplessness and in a state of internal flux by being told sex was evil and by having so many of their unanswered questions left to their imaginations.

There were opportunities, however, for boys and girls to socialize and flirt with each other. It might be nothing more than young men having the opportunity to walk young women home from church through the woods with the parents usually not too far behind. Sure, these young people did experience sexual feelings, feeling feisty and horny sometimes, but they were often left feeling guilty because they were taught that these thoughts were sinful and dirty.

What did the spiritual leaders of the day have to say about all this? There are those who may agree or disagree that the church often did more to confuse children concerning the subject of sex than anything else. Of course, the church has the Holy Bible as its guide, and I certainly do not argue this fact. The church when we were growing up did not touch the subject much, except that the preacher would preach against such sins as fornication and adultery. The church, otherwise, left the subject to the wisdom of the parents. There were no sex education classes for young people in either school or church. So, all in all, the children got very few details concerning human sexuality. There was an educational void in this area of life. Our parents did the very best they could with what they had been given by the generations before them. Our own generation continues to wrestle with such issues today. At least the problem is being brought to the surface, and the debate is lively!

Minnie Came by It Honestly

Minnie Jones was born in miserable and unpromising conditions. She grew up as a Negro, as a girl, economically poor, and in the heart of Southern racism and sexism. Her life was a struggle against the odds right from the beginning. Her early childhood was spent in a predominantly Negro, segregated environment. To an extent, however, we were sheltered from the most overt racial discrimination of the time. Both our maternal and paternal grandparents were landowners, which gave them some status in the community.

While our family basically subsisted in abject poverty, in many ways we were rich. We had two parents in the home. Throughout our parents' entire marriage, only once did our mother threaten to leave Daddy. She did go to Detroit and stay a while with our sister Katie. Momma and Daddy worked out whatever the trouble was, and the two remain together at this writing. Both are aging and in poor health today, but, thank God, we still have them both and they have always been there for us.

Our family had the blessing of strong support from our grandparents and others in the community, as well. Both our parents had some education and had great respect for learning and family life. Our parents were able to instill strong spiritual values in us. Our parents belonged to Tabernacle Christian Methodist Episcopal Church as we grew up, and they remain members today. Momma was always actively involved in church activities. We were kept active in Sunday School and religious education classes, and we attended church singing conventions, picnics and dinners-on-the-ground, etc. The old saying, sometimes attributed to Abraham Lincoln, is right, "No [one] is poor who has had a Godly mother." On the one hand it is remarkable that such humble beginnings could have produced the kind of achievers which the offspring of Haller and Curtis Jones have become. On the other hand, our parents gave us all the ingredients we needed to succeed in life and how could we have done anything less.

Minnie Jones went on to become the best known of the Jones family. But those of us who were close to her in the early years know her belief that success requires sacrifice. She was willing to sacrifice.

Momma recalls that Minnie didn't play very much, although she would play rag ball and a few other childhood games. Most often, she would find something to read and curl up in bed with it. She would read anything she could find: old textbooks, fairy tales, old almanacs, catalogs, the Bible, whatever was available At night when the oil lamp went down, she would place pine tree branches into the fireplace to give her enough light to enable her to continue her reading.

Of course, no one really recognized it at the time, but Little Minnie did exhibit an early interest in medicine and health-related concerns. She was inquisitive about the ingredients of such medicines and home remedies as 666 Cold Preparation; SSS Tonic, good for chills and fever; Black Draught; and cow chip tea made by taking dry cow dung tied in a rag, steeping it in hot water and adding turpentine, pine needles, red onion and horehound. Momma recounts that "*Minnie's little head was always filled with curiosity for how to cure and save lives. She was always fond of dogs and cats and took time to examine their teeth and check them over for fleas and ticks.*" She also spent time just daydreaming. About what? She is the only one who really knows.

Because she was always a fast learner and a good pupil, Minnie excelled as a student. The payoff for her academic excellence began early in her life. By age fifteen, she had worked her way through the twelve grade county school. Her future plans were uncertain at that point, because scholarships were not readily available for Negro students, and outside their own families there was little encouragement for them to go to college. But, "where there is a will, there is a way!"

The Jones family, like most Negro families at that time, faced first poverty and second racial discrimination. While these conditions were indeed obstacles, they did not keep Minnie from having a happy childhood. Although she was poor, she never considered herself poor. It didn't matter that she was born and reared in a shotgun shack without the comfort of modern conveniences. She felt wealthy! Richness in love, hope, self-esteem, determination, along with spiritual values, moral values and a strong work ethic, were somehow given to the Jones children by Haller and Curtis Jones. It was against this backdrop that the doctor, who in 1992 would become America's "top doctor," would begin to emerge.

A Long Way from Schaal

It may seem unlikely that these humble beginnings would produce the United States Surgeon General. It is a long way from Schaal to Washington. It is like the old story about the elderly lady in rural Southwest Arkansas who was stopped one Sunday morning while walking to church. The person who stopped her was from the Governor's office and asked directions to get to Schaal. The lady is reported to have said, *"If I had wanted to get there, I sure wouldn't have started here."* None of us get to choose our own starting place. Dr. Elders didn't. And most of us could probably find a better place than where we started from. However, since it is not ours to choose, we must simply roll up our sleeves and go to work to make a better future for ourselves.

Chapter Three

FROM THE HOG PEN TO THE WASHPOT: SOUTHERN BLACK COMMUNITY RITUALS THAT LI'L MINNIE KNEW

The Role of Rituals

Rituals are more caught than taught, you learn them by participation, not by information. They were the community's credo. It was what we believed. The dance was ritualistic/traditional. All these rules were learned at an early age and we were not always aware we were being taught. A ritual is the established form for a religious or community ceremony. The ritual is performed under a prescribed set of circumstances and pervades the whole of the community's life. It is like when I was in the Army. I had to salute the commissioned officers in appropriate circumstances. Saluting in the Army is a ritual. It is as much a part of Army life as saying "good morning" to every person you would meet when Li'l Minnie was growing up in rural Southwest Arkansas. A person could have participated in a Ku Klux Klan ritual the night before, but if you walked by that person on the road the next day, he had to speak to you. The Southern community ritual required it. If you did not follow the prescribed and established ritual of greeting everyone you met on the road or trail, you could almost be arrested. It had nothing to do with race or color; it had to do with the established community ritual. Saying "good morning" was a cardinal virtue.

We all know that a ritual has special importance for religious ceremonies like baptizing babies, wedding ceremonies and funerals. But I contend the ritual was very much a part of every aspect of Southern black community life.

There are many ritual acts in Christianity, such as: laying on hands to signify the transmission of an office and kneeling in prayer to show reverence.

Many of the Southern black community rituals have been abolished altogether. There are many different opinions about the value of rituals and ceremonies. The ritual says there are things we just know. We don't know how we know, we just know. The rituals equip us to turn positive everyday habits into a sense of reverence and mutual respect.

Rituals unite the interests and objectives of the community into a desire to define and pass on the cultural heritage that identifies the community itself. Rituals are the most important element in identifying the common history of a community.

Family Roots, Folklore, and Cultural Heritage

Rituals say only those who are born here and marry someone who was born here can be full members of the community. If you were not born or married into a rural Southern black church you can join and participate for sixty years and not be recognized as an "official" member. There is no other way to become a full member of a small rural community or black church except to be born into it.

Rituals are a repository of creative expressions that bear witness to the freedom of expression in the life of Li'l Minnie. Rituals are a part of the common history of most black Americans born before the Korean War and the great migration from the South. Rituals help to foster the continuation of an unshakable adherence to tradition. Indeed, most of these rituals are no longer a way of life for black Americans. However, I contend there is a storehouse of learning in the infinite variety of Southern rituals practiced during the early childhood of Li'l Minnie. Certainly the experiences our family had were not unique to us; we practiced the same sorts of rituals that many families did back then. These rituals were passed down from generation to generation. It is up to us to keep the rituals and traditions alive and to keep passing them on—perhaps if not the actual ritual acts performed, then at least we can keep the stories alive. We must do this through our families. The family is the most important force in the life of every individual. We can trace our family roots in Southern Arkansas back four generations. Li'l Minnie's' family "roots" ordained her as a part of the last generation that will serve as historian of these community rituals (who actually participated in the rituals). That is why it is so compelling and relevant to include them in this book. Knowing something about our family's past is of anthropological value in understanding the plight of black Americans in their will to survive in the days of segregation, Jim Crow and racism. Unless we understand this part of America's history, we are condemned to repeat the past in order to learn that black Americans are not strangers in this country—even though a majority of black Americans still often feel strange, and like strangers in a strange land. Although my family roots go back farther and are deeper than many white Americans, I feel like a stranger at times, because I still have to prove that I am a native American.

Rituals help to understand and define the ongoing nature of Southern black life in rural Southwest Arkansas during Li'l Minnie's' childhood. These rituals ranged in a variety of styles from the casual Sunday dinner to the dressed re-enactment of a Thanksgiving dinner, with a fixed time, place and script. A significant moment was when Grandma would pray thanking God for every blessing we received, didn't receive and should have received. By the time she was through Grandpa would ask her to re-heat the giblet gravy for the turkey. These special meals were immortalized through rituals and customs.

There is no zeal in my family for reliving the past. There is, however, zeal to revisit some of the places and share some of the events that helped to shape the life of this crusading Southern black woman. There is a fervent solidarity on the part of my family to tell our story. The story of Dr. M. Joycelyn Elders has been mis-told by almost every newspaper, radio and television commentator in the country. Now it is time to tell our own story. "Our time under God is now." To God be the glory"!

The Hog Killing University Ritual

> *Your grandfather, Charlie Jones was the best hog-killer in the country.*
> William A. Dillard

Hog-killing was a community ritual that occurred in the late fall every year. People had to wait until the late fall when it was cool enough for the meat to keep without refrigeration. Our parents' home had no icebox or refrigerator until Joycelyn was in her second year of college. Our parents had a smoke house for the parts of the hog that could be smoked, salted down, dry cured and kept, such as hams, shoulders and sausage. The other part of the hog that had been butchered, such as the intestines (chitterlings), liver, mountain oysters, and tenderloins had to be divided up among the ritual participants and eaten the day, or within hours, of the slaughter. Often the people who had no hogs to kill would come and help others in the community kill their hogs. They would get the hog's head, the feet, and, in some cases, they would talk people out of such choice cuts as the liver or some spare ribs. But in most cases, the main cuts from the hog were used to bargain and trade with other people in the community whose hogs they would slaughter later in the fall. The fall was the best time, but not the only time, for butchering hogs because you needed several days of cool weather for adequate time to process the fresh meat and preserve it. Nothing is worse than a warm spell in the weather following the hog slaughtering ritual and losing a choice ham to flies and maggots. That is preferably why the best time for butchering a hog is when you can follow the *Farmer's Almanac* in predicting several days when the temperature will hover around 32 to 34 degrees. The two most used books, most of the time the only two books, in our parents' home were the Holy Bible and the *Farmer's Almanac*. The *Farmer's Almanac* was my parents' guide for predicting the weather before they had a radio or knew about the weatherman. Our parents would go over the *Farmer's Almanac* to find out when to butcher or castrate a hog, plant cotton, cut hay, or pull one of our loose teeth.

The Hog-Killing Preparation
─────────────────────────

The hog-killing preparation was an exciting family and community ritual when Li'l Minnie was growing up in rural Southwest Arkansas. The preparation involved planning, organizing and lots of family and community participation. There were times our father killed as many as three hogs on the same day.

In preparation for the slaughter, the hog spent his last month confined in a small pen eating corn and shorts and drinking all it could gobble down. The corn was fed to the hog because the grain made the hog's meat firmer and more tasty. For the most part, we would only feed our hogs dishwater slop, culled cucumbers, field weeds and watermelons during the summer and early fall. In preparing the hogs for the slaughter, all the little male pigs were castrated when they were six weeks old by my father and Minnie. Sometimes, however, it could be on the fifth week or as late as the seventh week depending on the *Farmer's Almanac*, the moon and the weather. My father always wanted to castrate the pigs during the day after the night of a half-moon. This tradition had something to do with the testicles (which we called mountain oysters) being in the shape of a half-moon. After the little pig was castrated, Minnie would take the testicles and put them in a water bucket and while our father was still holding the little pig, which was squealing for dear life, Katie would dress the cut down with creosote dip. The creosote dip was a kind of antiseptic made from coal tar and was used on all animal cuts to prevent infection and keep the flies from laying their eggs in the fresh wound causing maggots to hatch there. My flesh still crawls when I think about my sisters, Minnie and Katie, holding a little pig or shoat (small hog) while our father used a little branch from a tree as a scalpel to perform the surgery to remove the maggots out of the hog. Doctoring on animal cuts took a lot of work and a lot of our father's time during the summer months. The problem with flies was much less severe during the fall and winter.

Often after a day of castrating pigs, Minnie would have to clean a water bucket full of mountain oysters. For supper that night we all could eat as many mountain oysters as we wanted. As a young boy growing up my male friends had a rumor out that mountain oysters made one a real man, because you were taking on additional power from the little male pigs. However, as I grew older, I came to realize that if the mountain oysters could really give one so much additional power, then it would have helped to save all the pigs from ending up in the slaughter house.

The Day of Sacrifice

On the day of slaughter I often wondered if the hog knew that it was getting ready to meet its maker. I noticed that the behavior of the hog would at times seem to change. The squeal would turn into a litany of short grunts. On the day of the slaughter, Minnie, as the oldest child, would help our parents during the ritual by giving direction to a congregation of participants who had gathered. The hog-killing ceremony would start out with the rhythm and harmony of the Mormon Tabernacle Choir. Our family would start the ritual, under the direction of my mother and Minnie, on a cool frosty morning. Our whole family played a role in the entire ritual.

Rev. Frisk, our preacher was always present for the hog killings to say a prayer and get God's share of the meat. Sometimes Momma would remind him that Jesus was Jewish and did not eat pork. When Rev. Frisk was present, we would always start the killing ritual with prayer. My memory is somewhat faded, but as much as I can recall the prayer went something like:

> O Lord, we are thankful that you have blessed us today with good hog killing weather. Bless this time as we come together to butcher these hogs. We pray for the forgiveness of our sins of omission and commission. We pray for every lost sinner in Howard County. We thank you, O Lord, for the sacrifice you made of your Son, our Lord and Savior, even Jesus Christ, for the sins of the whole world.
> Now Lord! Now Lord! Forgive us as we help Brother Curtis and Haller butcher these hogs so that our tables may be blessed with food to nourish our bodies with physical strength to do your will for our salvation and your glory. This we pray in the name of Jesus. Amen.

Then the two older boys were detailed to make a fire around the washpot. The washpot was filled with water from the rain barrel and a hot fire was made around it to bring the water to a scalding boil. The washpot was made of cast iron to withstand the heat. The washpot was heated by dry pine kindling and dry limbs that would burn fast and hot.

When the water was boiling and scalding hot, our father was informed and would swing into action. The hog pen was only about one quarter of a mile away from the house. Our father would take his single shot 22 caliber rifle to the hog pen and death would come quickly for the hog with the crack of that gun.

After the shot, our father would use a long sharp knife to stab the hog under the throat, between the two front shoulder blades, near the heart, in order to get a good bleed from the hog. The hog's blood would gush out like water from a burst water line, first spurting out fast, then slowing down and becoming thick and lumpy. This process is where the old saying, "bleeding like a stuck pig" comes from. The pig, in some cases after being stuck, would stagger to its feet for a brief moment, but usually death came instantly.

The hog pen was far enough away from the house that our father had to use our horse, old Dick, to drag the hog up to the wash place where the hog could be scalded in a 55 gallon barrel that was set on an angle, tilted back, in the ground. The hog was always scalded head first, because that was the most difficult part to clean the hair from. If the water temperature was right the hair could be peeled off with your hands. In most cases, the hog would be dunked in and out of the barrel two or three times. After the hog was fairly clean of hog hair a singletree, or a strong stick, was used to hoist the hog up by the tendons in the hind legs. A large hog had to be lifted up with a block-in-line hanging from a strong limb on the gum tree by the house. The hog was lifted until its head cleared the ground. After the hog was hoisted up and hanging from the tree more scalding water was poured over the hog and it was scraped until the skin was clear of hog hair.

When the hog was washed down and cleaned, our father would make a slit and open the hog's belly so that the intestines and stomach would fall into a #3 galvanized washtub that had been placed under it. After the intestines and stomach were removed, a cut was made around the hog's head and it was taken off. The hog was then cut in half, taken down and placed on the wash bench where the final cuts were made and the meat was taken to the smokehouse. The hog was cut into many sections and parts with a meat cleaver. The cleaver and knife were used to cut out the fat from the back bone for lard, and the tenderloin was used for making sausage. The sausage was made with a meat grinder. It was seasoned with red pepper, black pepper and sage. The sage was roasted in the kitchen stove until dry, put in a rag and beaten up and sprinkled in the sausage. The lard was made from the fat on the hog which was taken and boiled in a washpot until the fat bellies would turn into cracklin's, or fried pork skins. After the leaf of fat was cut out, the middlin', or bacon, was left to be salted down, along with the hams and shoulders. The hams and shoulders were hung in the smokehouse and smoked for days with hickory and sassafras until they were cured.

The hog's head would be cleaned, split open and the brain was removed to cook with scrambled eggs for breakfast. Sometimes we would make hog head cheese from the hog's head and other parts.

The hog's intestines and stomach were taken and washed and cleaned a number of times and then cooked and called chitterlings. Often the hog's melt would be cooked in the ashes around the washpot or in the fireplace. The average hog, according to our father's father, would produce about ten pounds of chitterlings per hundred weight, including the stomach. It was always Minnie's job to clean and cook the stomach. It was always Minnie's job to clean and cook the chitterlings. Even now I feel that my sister cooked some of the best chitterlings in the world. She probably would still be Surgeon General if she had spent more time cooking and serving chitterlings to the politicians on Capitol Hill, after all, they are partial to "pork bellies."

Chitterlings were always a regular part of our family's diet. Chitterlings were thrown away by most white folks until they found out we were eating them. On Thanksgiving day when we had my grandparents and other relatives over for dinner Minnie would cook our chitterlings in the washpot outside. The washpot was the hub of many activities on the farm before the arrival of modern-day conveniences. The washpot was smooth as a new born baby's skin on the inside, and black and rough as an alligator's hide on the outside. The washpot had three cow-teat-like legs that it stood on and was always placed on three bricks to elevate it. The washpot was made of cast-iron and could withstand almost any amount of heat. The pot was often heated by pine kindling and dry wood or anything that would start quick and burn fast. The washpot served many functions such as: boiling water for killing hogs, cooking lard from the fat off a large hog, making lye soap, boiling the dirt out of clothes, etc.

Making Cracklings

Cracklings were made from the fat belly of a large hog. The fat belly was cut into small cubes and cooked in the washpot. The fat on the skin of the hog's belly would be cooked and turned into hot grease. After the grease would cool down it would turn white and was called lard. The lard was taken out of the washpot and put in a five gallon lard can. Lard was used for everything from frying eggs to frying fish and rabbit. All farm families in the South in the early forties and fifties have memories of cooking lard and making cracklings, or porkrinds.

When the cubes from the fat belly were ready they would turn into cracklings, crisp and dry. and would rise to the top of the washpot. A large strainer was used when they were ready to dip them out and the lard was poured into a lard bucket after it had cooled down. It was then stored in the smokehouse. We cooked everything in lard in those days because we had never heard about calories and cholesterol.

The washpot was used to make lye soap. The lye soap was often made from sick animals on the farm that had died. The animal would be dragged up to the wash place, cut up, placed into the washpot where a fire was made to cook it down. The soap was made from wood ashes and red devil lye. The lye came in a small soup can sized container with the picture of a red devil with his pitchfork and tail working over a red hot flame. Lye soap was used to wash clothes and to bathe with when we had no store-bought soap. When the soap was ready it would turn tan.

Wash Day

Wednesday was always wash day at our parents' home. Somehow our mother felt that this was the only day God made for washing all the family's clothes. It was the only day our mother felt you could get the clothes really clean.

Washing, before the days of washing machines, was done on a scrub-board. Bleach was used to help get the clothes clean. Often the washpot was filled with rain water caught in a barrel where it ran off the house after a rain. The barrel was left in that place all the time.

On wash day Minnie would help our mother stir, punch and poke the clothes with the handle from an old, worn-out broom.

Hog Pen Sex Education Down on the Farm

When the boar and the sow were courting we could watch them in action. But we could not let our parents catch us looking directly at the hogs when they were breeding. Our father always felt it was a taboo, a "no-no" to watch the hogs during such an intimate act. After all, the hogs, like humans, wanted and needed their privacy. The experience was not much different from that of humans. The boar would sometimes spend hours, or even days, in a foreplay-like manner with the sow before a sex act started. I have known and watched cases when a sow played "hard to get" and the boar's foreplay went on for as much as a week. The boar would use his snout to rub, touch and play with every area of the sow's body. In some cases, this was a real Romeo and Juliet act. The courting went on and on until the grunting and squalling became a love song. Unlike women, sows cannot be raped, rushed or forced into a sex act. For the sow the act of mating is never a pleasure. It is always for reproduction. The litter of piglets produced from the act of mating is usually from six to nine. However, a good sow can, in some cases, have as many as eighteen to twenty piglets in a litter. However, a large litter like that is an exception, much like our maternal grandmother giving birth to eighteen children.

When the sow is finally worked up and ready, the breeding starts. If someone brought a sow to be bred by our father's boar and they tried to wait around for the mating to take place we children were told to go to the house or up in the field and play.

One of the things that you must keep in mind is that hogs behave much like humans. I noticed a considerable difference between how the boar related to a sow that was brought to be bred, over against how the boar related to a sow that was a part of the hog pen family he knew and sow that was a part of the hog pen family he knew and considered to be one of his "hogfriends" or "hogwives." In almost all of these relationships the boar spent a great deal of time in foreplay and in building up the relationship, or so it seemed. Whereas, with a sow the boar considered to be a stranger, or something like a prostitute, the meeting seemed to be no more than a man going to a prostitute. In this instance the act was just a case of "blim, blam, thank you ma'am." But when the boar had to deal with one of his "hogwives," the relationship was different than it was when it was breeding with strange hogs. When our father was not around I would watch the breeding along with my cousins, J.D. and Tunk. We would take turns watching and standing lookout for our parents. We were enthralled by the gristle-like object of the boar slipping in and out in a bracing bite-like action until the point of climax when the sow would cry out in a loud scream and the boar would let out a final grunt of relief and crawl down. If the squalling took place about the same time you knew that you stood a good chance that conception had taken place. At this point, the sow would walk around for a while and the boar, just like a man, would go to the mudhole and wallow a couple of times and go to sleep. Some people say boys and girls from the country make all around better husbands and wives because they learn about sex education from the way animals related to one another, rather than watching a movie made in Hollywood. Most of us who grew up on the farm can testify to the fact that we have never seen a sow raped, abused, or forced into the sex act. I have never seen, or heard, any animals having sex simply for pleasure. Their acts are always to replenish the earth. This is a lesson that all of us modern day humans could use in teaching our youngsters about family values.

Chapter Four

WINTER SUNSET

*And not only so, but we glory in tribulations also;
knowing that tribulation worketh patience;
and patience, experience; and experience, hope. . .*
(Romans 5:3-4 KJV)

Glory in Tribulation
―――――――――――――

If we are to understand what this passage of scripture really means, we should learn to appreciate, rather than decry, our trials in life. Although she may not have fully understood it at the time, Joycelyn learned very early in her life that "we also rejoice in our sufferings, because we know that suffering produces perseverance, perseverance, character, and character hope." (Romans 5:3-4 NIV)

In addition, we understand that God speaks to us through various media. But to find direction and inspiration in what is communicated to us, we must be tuned in to His presence and hear Him. Such an experience almost always leaves a lasting impression on us. We feel differently, and so we act differently. Joycelyn feels she had such a divine encounter through the medium of a high school play in which she participated. The play was entitled *Winter Sunset.* This play, and the events leading up to it are crucial in understanding who Joycelyn Elders is.

California Days
―――――――――――

Momma and Daddy moved to California in 1943. They brought Joycelyn along as the baby-sitter for me while they worked in the shipyards. Our sister Katie and the older boys, Charles and Bernard, remained behind in Schaal with our grandparents, because our maternal grandfather did not want anything to happen to Charles, who was his namesake and favorite grandson. Three of our siblings were therefore left behind but were expected to join us later, when Momma and Daddy were established and had a place for all of us to live.

When we arrived in California, we stayed with our cousins in Richmond at 1361 Kelsey Street. Our cousins had a large place they had renovated into a rooming house with apartments for rent to the many relatives who were leaving the farm and moving to California to work in the shipyards during World War II. The cousins with whom we lived were Beryl and Charlie Reid and their children Ivey, Florence and Charlie, Jr. They had moved to California with the first wave of sharecroppers who had left the South during the Depression. Beryl and Charlie, in particular, had been able to find work and, for Negroes of that time, were doing quite well economically. They had worked in the shipyards and factories, pooled their money and purchased the large rooming house located on the edge of the city limits of Richmond.

When the second large wave of rural Negroes looking for work migrated to California from Arkansas, Louisiana and Texas, the public schools could not accommodate all of the children. To address the overcrowding, the school day had to be divided into two shifts. The first shift, or class day, ended at 1:30 p.m. This schedule was helpful to many families in which the older children had to keep their younger siblings until their parents returned home from a shift change. The arrangement worked out well for me, because it meant that Joycelyn only had to baby-sit me for two and one half hours after school, until Momma came home from working the day shift. Daddy kept me in the morning while Momma worked and Joycelyn was in school.

Since so many of the Negro children had come from sharecropping families in the South, many of them could not read or write, even though they might have reached the eighth or ninth grade. So, all the children coming to California to enroll in school had to be tested to determine their grade placement. Many children were placed back a number of grades before they could enroll in the California school system. This was so embarrassing for some children that they decided to go back to the rural South to continue their education in the segregated Southern schools.

Joycelyn, however, tested at two grade levels above the rest of her class and her age level. Since she had started school at five years of age, a compromise was reached with our parents, and she ended up being advanced only one grade.

Joycelyn enjoyed California. She did well in school and loved living away from the farm in rural Arkansas—if only for a few years. She loved the huge grape harvest and the big garden out back of the house. (She is an avid gardener today.) The cousins with whom we lived also raised and sold rabbits. As it turned out, the West Coast experience was a good one for her. It was not surprising that once the war ended and our parents lost their jobs in the shipyards and decided to return to Schaal, Joycelyn wanted to stay in California. Our parents, of course, could not grant her wish.

Back to the Farm

Many Negroes were unable to find jobs after the war and had to move back to the rural South to start life as sharecroppers all over again. Despite having her hopes of staying in California dashed, Joycelyn was always thankful for the education she received while in the California school system. Indeed, something about the California experience seemed to prepare her for the return to life in rural Arkansas.

Young people, especially those in their early teens, seem to have a difficult time understanding why their parents sometimes have to pick up and move, taking the youngsters from what seems to be a dream come true-in Joycelyn's case, friends and a good school system that offered a life filled with dreams, hope, love and vision. Even today, when parents must move for economic reasons, many children have a difficult time making the adjustment, sometimes to the point of becoming depressed enough to take their own lives. There are also those who make the adjustment and go on with their lives.

(In my opinion, parents should be more sensitive and take into consideration the possible impact that a radical move may have on their children, especially teenagers in their "salad and dressing years"—ages 13-16. It may be good to bring the children who are mature enough into the decision-making process.)

Nevertheless, in our family situation at the time, coming back to Arkansas was probably good for all concerned. Joycelyn had no way of knowing at the time that God may have had a hand in the event: had she not returned, she could not have readied herself for President Bill Clinton's call.

When Joycelyn returned to Arkansas, she made the adjustment and was enrolled in the ninth grade at Howard County Training School. Her last three years of high school were spent studying, participating in debate groups, speaking bees, spelling matches, playing roles in school plays and reading poetry. As a child, Joycelyn had learned to memorize long passages by reading the same books over and over again. She has never lost this knack. Even today, she memorizes most of her speeches and can quote names, numbers, and other statistical data without the aid of notes or script.

Art: Poetry and Drama

Not many know that she is an artful reader of poetry. Her favorite reading is still "If" by Rudyard Kipling. I attended a reading she gave for a group at the Little Rock Public Library a few years ago during Black History Week. I found she would be reading that particular day through a public announcement carried in the Arkansas Democrat newspaper. To tell the truth, I did not want to go with her, because I had never really heard my sister read serious poetry before. So, I slipped in the back door after the reading had started, in order not to be embarrassed by being identified with a person who I felt had no strong ability at poetry reading, and one who would surely make a fool of herself before a large crowd.

I was astonished at what I heard. She warmed the crowd up that day by reading some of Paul Lawrence Dunbar's poems and Tennyson's "Crossing the Bar," but she finished up by bringing the crowd to its feet when she read "If." I thought, "That poem was made for her."

When she had finished, I joined the standing ovation. In fact, I was so moved that I left my seat and rushed down to stand with her because I was proud and wanted to be identified with her.

In our many conversations around the dinner table, or working on a piece of property, or just riding together in the car for a visit with our parents, Joycelyn and I have often recapitulated our childhood days. It is not very often, however, that I am able to catch my sister in a moment where she is reminiscent about her youth. It is real work to create a climate in which she will share much about her thoughts concerning her early life—even with her younger brother. But on a few occasions I have persuaded her to share bits and pieces with me.

Once, she shared with me that one of her most memorable and life-impacting experiences was her participation in the school play, *Winter Sunset*. It helped her after returning from California to understand the plight of sharecroppers, and it served to lift her spirit and give her hope. Joycelyn recalled for me what the play was about. In actuality the play was not one which focused on a very hopeful theme. *Winter Sunset* was a play which told the story of a young couple in Kansas trying to survive as wheat farmers. One year, with a good wheat crop in the fields just before the harvest, the fields caught fire and everything was lost. The rest of the story centered around how this young couple faced this tragedy and struggled to make it through the long harsh winter. In the final scene, when winter was almost over, and the family had survived, there was a beautiful winter sunset in which spring, with its promise of new hope, could be discerned.

The play also showed how the coldness of winter can affect our moods. Dreary cold days can keep us bound inside and perhaps give us "cabin fever." But winter can also be a wonderful time of the year: it is a time to read good books; it is an opportunity to spend more time with the family and just do fun things. Winter doesn't have to be depressing. We can use the winter to reflect, and plan for the "winter sunset" and the coming of spring. The question we need to ask ourselves during the winter, while we wait, is not "why did this happen to me," but "what is the promise hidden in this event." We can see the coming "winter sunset" if we remember to anticipate it.

Life Imitates Art

There have been many "winter sunset" experiences in Joycelyn's life. She shared with me one of the more unforgettable ones which occurred during her confirmation process. The long and controversy-filled hearings were for Joycelyn the "winter sunset" before the "spring" of her confirmation as Surgeon General. This particular experience came when the Senator from Kansas, Nancy Kassebaum, offered the following statement on the Senate floor:

> Whatever doubt there may be about Dr. Elders as the messenger, there can be no doubt about the importance of her message. Teenage pregnancy is a serious and growing problem, and we face a grim future indeed if it is not addressed. Dealing with this issue has proved to be a baffling and frustrating task. It is tragic that far too many parents have shirked their responsibility to guide and discipline their children. There simply is no satisfactory substitute for strong parenting in terms of instilling the values and the hope which inspire responsible behavior by young people.
>
> The sad reality is that many young people do not or cannot rely on the support and guidance of their parents. Dr. Elders is faced with that reality. She has attempted to deal with that reality by sending loud, clear, and yes—flamboyant messages. However uncomfortable I or other members of this body may be with her words, I believe she should be heard. She deserves the chance to try to reach young people whom no one else seems to be able to reach. In the final analysis, my decision to support Dr. Elders' nomination was based on the hope that she will be able to strike a chord with young

people whom I could never dream of reaching....

Finally, Dr. Elders is a hard worker who understands firsthand many of the public health challenges confronting our Nation. I will join those voting in favor of her nomination. I will do so in hope that she can convey a message which will be heard by young people making critical decisions about their futures. (U.S. Cong. Joint Committee on Printing S11006-S11007)

While Senator Kassebaum's words represented a "winter sunset" in the confirmation process for Joycelyn, her words may also be interpreted as a "winter sunset" for Americans. Joycelyn dared to stand tall and give recognition to the fact that teenage pregnancy is a serious and growing problem, and our future will be grim if the problem continues to go unchecked.

Senator Kassebaum dared to pull back the cover on the fact that too many young people do not, and can not, rely on the support and guidance of their parents. She had the guts to give her unequivocal support to Joycelyn, the controversial but realistic messenger. At the same time, when Senator Kassebaum concluded that her decision to support Joycelyn's nomination was based on the hope that she would be able to strike a chord with young people she could never dream of reaching, it was a "winter sunset" for young people, too.

I wonder how many of America's young people can identify with the scene? We need more Nancy Kassebaums who will help Americans survive these long, dark, dreary days of winter: the vestiges of racial and sexist hate; injustice; the mistreatment of the poor; crime; and mean-spirited attempts to repress hope in too many of the people.

We need a "winter sunset" in our country. We need hope for our children and for ourselves. This hope is what Dr. Elders is about. She learned through the experiences of her life about the importance of hope—about the importance of knowing that winter will end and spring will come. Dr. Elders is doing her share, all she can, to help us move toward that "winter sunset."

Chapter Five

THE FIRST LEG OF A LONG JOURNEY

"Let Down Your Bucket"

Minnie graduated from Howard County Training School in Tollette, Arkansas in May of 1949 at the tender age of 15. She was the valedictorian of her class, despite the many days she had to miss school to help our family on the farm picking and chopping cotton. In her valedictory speech to her class, her message was, "Let Down Your Bucket Where You Are."

She received the inspiration for this address, in part, from reading about the life of Booker T. Washington. There is a story attributed to Washington about a ship that was lost at sea. The captain sent a signal, "water, water, we die of thirst." And the answer came, "Cast down your bucket where you are" (Johnson 325). And, in part, Minnie's speech was inspired by something our paternal grandmother (for whom she was named) said to her on one occasion when she had sent Minnie to draw water from the well that Grandpa and Daddy had dug. Minnie had tried to stand in the same place our grandmother had stood while drawing water, but that particular place was wet and muddy. So she had moved to another spot around the well, and she was not sure the pulley and rope on the well could let the bucket down from where she was standing. Her indecision had taken too much time and our grandmother came out of the kitchen and asked, "Minnie, what in the world is taking you so long?" "I am trying to find a place to draw the water, where I won't get my shoes muddy," she replied. By now, our grandmother's patience had grown thin because she needed some water for the pinto beans cooking on the kitchen stove. "Let down your bucket where you are!" she commanded.

The advice from our grandmother became a lifelong philosophy of little Minnie Lee Jones from Schaal. Having a desire to draw water from the well of higher education, she let down her bucket where she was, and her desires and prayers were answered. She received a scholarship to Philander Smith College, a predominantly black college in Little Rock, Arkansas related to the Methodist Church. The Scholarship was awarded by a group of Methodist women who recognized her gifts and accomplishments.

College Bound

The summer of 1949 was a long, hot one for Minnie. The anxiety of just thinking about being away from home and family for the first time was not easy. The summer was spent in preparation for college at Philander Smith. Minnie's preparation was most difficult because she had no one in her family with whom she could talk about college life; none of them had ever completed a college education.

At the end of August it was time to leave for school, and Momma asked Daddy to give Minnie some money for her bus fare to Little Rock. He told her he did not have the money.

At this point the real motivation for Minnie to get a college education came from Momma. Daddy, like most black men of that time, was struggling to provide for his family, and he could see little value in his oldest daughter going to college. The lot fell upon Momma to find the money to get Minnie to Philander.

I have raised the question with my mother and my sister, "Why, after having a whole summer to save money for college, did you not have enough money saved for a Greyhound bus ticket to Little Rock?" I realize, however, that in 1995 I am raising that question from the perspective of one who has a steady income and no children. No one who has not been in the position of a poor black sharecropping family in rural Southwest Arkansas in 1949 could even come close to understanding how this happened. Today we think of $3.50 for a one-way bus ticket to Little Rock as something you could pick up off the ground. But it was not so for a family of ten back then in rural Arkansas, where most black families had no savings and lived each day "from hand to mouth." My parents, out of necessity, had to live "just one day at a time." My mother has always lived her life by her faith that "the Lord will make a way somehow." And the Lord did, with the help of Minnie's mother, brothers and sisters. We had to go to the cotton field and scrap enough early cotton to buy Minnie a bus ticket. This chore was a major project for the family, and it took a couple of days. The cotton was sold to Fred Jones for $5.00. That sale proved to be a watershed in Minnie's life.

Uncle Slim, who had a truck, took us all, except our father, to Nashville, Arkansas, where Minnie got on the bus and waved good-bye to us. When the bus took off, Momma started to cry, and we all cried all the way home.

A freshman in college at fifteen, Minnie embarked on her life-changing mission. She changed her name to M. Joycelyn, taking on her own name and identity. She had found the name "Joycelyn" on the wrapper of her favorite peppermint candy.

Joycelyn never felt ashamed of who she was, or her economic and material shortcomings. When she arrived at Philander, arrangements had been made for her to live in the private home of a Little Rock family and work as a live-in maid in order to help pay her tuition. She cleaned, cooked, washed clothing, mopped floors and performed other domestic chores. She never resented her work as a "domestic engineer," because she thought hard work was a way of life. Between her studies and her domestic chores, Joycelyn attended very few social functions such as athletic games, picnics and dances. She did meet a young man at Philander, but their relationship never became serious. She had little time for socializing, and even less for romance.

Chapter Six

HEROES

<u>Determination Pays Off</u>

During her sophomore year at Philander Smith, Joycelyn's insatiable desire for learning was intensified by the encouragement of her biology instructor, Dr. J. D. Scott. Dr. Scott recognized her potential and encouraged her to reach for the sky.

College tuition costs increased Joycelyn's second year, placing a heavier financial burden on her and our family. At one point she had no money left to buy anything at all. Her only good pair of shoes had holes in them, and the sole on her right shoe had come loose. In desperation, Joycelyn wrote home to our mother for enough money to buy a pair of shoes. This request was very difficult for her to make, because she knew our parents were unlikely to be able to help. Since our parents had not expected their daughter to attend college, no preparations had been made to deal with emergencies like the need for a new pair of shoes.

After not hearing from Momma for two weeks, Joycelyn wrote another letter explaining the urgency of getting a new pair of shoes. Joycelyn was on the debating team and had won the prize for oratory for her class. She would therefore be on the debating team that traveled around the state competing with other college teams. She needed a decent pair of shoes to participate on the team.

Even though our mother was in bed pregnant with her youngest child, she asked God to give her the strength to walk up to Fred Jones' cotton field to scrap enough cotton to buy her daughter some shoes. My next oldest sister, Katie, and two older brothers, Bernard and Charles, had gone with my father down to the bottom farm to cut and shock hay. That left my mother, pregnant and with another baby, Pat, in her arms, along with me and my sister Beryl to pick the cotton. We picked 150 pounds of cotton to make the $3.75 to buy shoes for Joycelyn.

Before the money could be sent, Joycelyn was at the point of despair because of the financial burden she had placed on our parents and on us, her younger brothers and sisters. It was tough going for a sixteen-year-old to realize she had run out of money, food and school supplies, and had no way to get enough money to buy a pair of shoes.

On Friday of that week, Joycelyn went to see Dr. Scott to tell him she did not think she could take it anymore and had decided to drop out of college. Dr. Scott listened for a while to her story about being unable to go to classes hungry and with no shoes to wear. After she had poured out all of her problems, Dr. Scott said to her, "So what are you going to do when you drop out of college and go back home?" After some moments of silence, Dr. Scott said, "Well, I guess you will probably go back home to picking and chopping cotton again. But I know you are not a quitter. And your family did not send you up here to drop out and come back home." Dr. Scott went on with his pep talk to tell Joycelyn, "You are not in college just to represent yourself, you are here representing generations of family members and relatives who never had a chance to go to college. You must show your other brothers and sister that you are not a quitter. So, you can drop out and quit school if you want to. But as long as you want to stay here, you will be able to eat and sleep, and we are not going to put you out." He told Joycelyn to think about it over the weekend and talk with him again on Monday.

On Saturday Joycelyn received a letter from our mother with $6.00 to buy a pair of shoes, the $3.75 from the 150 pounds of cotton and $2.25 from our grandmother Minnie. On Monday, Joycelyn was back in school and ready for Dr. Scott's biology class.

An Impossible Dream?

It was also during Joycelyn's sophomore year that her life's purpose began to become clear to her. It was during a lecture to the Pyramid Club at Philander Smith while Joycelyn was in the process of pledging Delta Sigma Theta Sorority that she first knew that a woman could aspire to become a physician. Before going to college she had never even seen a physician. *"In the country, unless you're sick and dying, you don't go to the doctor. The public nurses would come to school and we would line up for the vaccinations, vision checks and things like that. So after hearing this internist speak to our Pyramid Club, I decided that I wanted to be just like her,"* she says (Blount 15). "I've said frequently that 'you can't be what you can't see, so if I'd never seen a doctor, how could I ever think I would ever be a doctor? And to be the surgeon general — I had never even heard of a surgeon general" (Russell 24). So, as a result of the Pyramid Club lecture by Dr. Edith Irby Jones (then a first year medical student and later the first black doctor to graduate from the University of Arkansas Medical School) Joycelyn knew with certainty what her mission in life would be. Joycelyn was able to meet with Dr. Jones after the lecture. Joycelyn has said of Dr. Jones' lecture, *"She talked about the difference between taking the high roads and the low roads, and I was just enchanted with her speech..."* (Russell p 24). Following the meeting Joycelyn never again took her eyes off the prize of finishing college and becoming a medical doctor. Before meeting Dr. Jones, Joycelyn had not met or received the services of a doctor before. After hearing her speak and meeting her, Joycelyn was determined to become "just like her." Dr. Jones, who is currently a physician in Houston, Texas, has been Dr. Elders' mentor and long-time friend. In Dr.

Jones' profession, Joycelyn found her niche.

Working Her Way Up

After her second year in college, Joycelyn went to Kansas City, Missouri to spend the summer with our Aunt Joella Sewell, and she worked in the homes of some white families. When the summer ended, she returned to Little Rock to start her third year at Philander Smith.

It was during that third year at Philander Smith that Joycelyn's favorite uncle, Dr. Tom, had been killed in an automobile accident in St. Paul, Minnesota. She experienced a deep sense of loss, loneliness and isolation. She felt isolated because our family did not have enough money to send her the $6.00 she needed for the round-trip bus ticket home to be with us at the time of the funeral. She received words of comfort in a letter from our mother, assuring her that all had gone well during the funeral and our uncle had gone on to join his earthly father who was in heaven with God. In a few weeks Joycelyn was able to begin adjusting to the death and finish her junior year.

At the end of the semester she returned home to work for the summer and to prepare for her senior year at Philander Smith. During the summer months Joycelyn worked chopping cotton, picking peaches and cucumbers, and doing other farm-related jobs. September arrived and Joycelyn returned to Little Rock for her final college year. Upon her return, the placement office informed her that a white supporter of the college, Eva Moore Morton, who resided in the Heights (an affluent section of the city), needed someone to work and live in her home. Joycelyn took the job. This experience proved to be a very positive one, and a life-long friendship developed between Joycelyn and Mrs. Morton. Mrs. Morton treated Joycelyn more like a daughter than a live-in maid.

Joycelyn's senior year proved to be very positive in many ways. She completed her requirements for graduation and ranked first in her class. Her triumph was tainted with disappointment, however, because no family members were able to attend the graduation ceremonies.

Chapter Seven

PATRIOT

Love, Marriage and War

During her senior year in college a romance developed between Joycelyn and Cornelius Reynolds. They met while both were students at Philander Smith; Cornelius was a year ahead of Joycelyn. He proposed to her, they became engaged, and they were married. After college he went to Milwaukee, Wisconsin and found a job as a teacher. Upon graduating from Philander, Joycelyn moved to Milwaukee to be with Cornelius and got a job as a lab technician in a Catholic hospital.

This experience with marriage and work was interrupted by the Korean War. After General MacArthur was fired by President Truman over his strategy for winning the war, many more Americans became aware for the first time that a real war was going on over there and not just a "police action." Joycelyn always seemed drawn to controversy, and this one was no exception. She considered MacArthur one of her military heroes. (I believe that one reason Joycelyn was so impressed with General MacArthur had to do with his Arkansas roots. While she was at Philander, she spent many hours in MacArthur Park, across the bridge and down the street from the college. MacArthur's birthplace is a museum in that park. I also find it ironic that MacArthur was fired by President Truman, just as Joycelyn was fired by President Clinton. I remember General MacArthur's speeches after he was fired and how he maintained his focus on that famous trinity, "duty, honor and country." I think Joycelyn has likewise kept her focus on these things. The call went out for women to support the war effort in Korea. Joycelyn answered the call in 1953 by enlisting in the Army as a WAC.

Joycelyn comes from a patriotic American family which watched eight of her uncles go to fight in World War II. At the time Joycelyn joined the WACs, she already had uncles in the service. One had been wounded in Korea and others were in the Army, some on the front line.

When Joycelyn enlisted in Milwaukee, she was sent to a base camp in Houston, Texas for her basic training and preparation to be a physical therapist. After completing her basic training in Texas she was assigned to Brooks Army Medical Hospital in Denver, Colorado.

Proud Patriot—Prouder Family

Joycelyn enjoyed her three years in service to her country. The experience was beneficial to her in many ways. Joycelyn received her commission as a second lieutenant and had a great experience in race relations. Although she was the only African-American in her unit, the experience was very positive.

During her service years, when Joycelyn would come home on leave, she would always buy our parents something special like a real icebox or, later on, our first television. It made us all very proud to have our big sister and role model home in her uniform. Even in the hot summer, when she was home on leave, we all wanted her to wear her uniform every day so people could see her. I was so proud of having a sister who was a lieutenant in the Army, I even wanted her to wear her uniform to the cotton patch to help us chop cotton. I remember one day when she got into a lovers' quarrel with my mother, because with the temperature at 95 degrees, my mother wanted her to wear her uniform when they went into Mineral Springs together. Joycelyn said it was too hot for the uniform, and not only Momma was disappointed, but the rest of us as well. In fact, when she decided not to wear her uniform, I decided not to go to town with them.

After serving at Brooks Army Medical Hospital for a year, Joycelyn was promoted to the rank of first lieutenant. She received an honorable discharge upon completing her three-year enlistment obligation.

When Joycelyn Came Marchin' Home

Following Joycelyn's discharge in 1956, she and Cornelius moved to Denver. They lived and worked there until she was accepted as a medical student back in Arkansas. The marriage soon ended. It may be that the strain of being in a military marriage for three years, together with the prospect of four years of medical school before starting a family, proved too much for the couple. It must be said, however, that they did not get a divorce because she went to medical school; they got a divorce because Cornelius came to the realization that Joycelyn would be a wonderful friend but not, by the traditional standards of the fifties, the sort of wife he wanted. Joycelyn and Cornelius mutually agreed to go their separate ways and are still friends today.

Chapter Eight

HER LIFE'S VOCATION

<u>A Dream Come True</u>

Joycelyn's military service gave her access to the G.I. Bill, which helped turn her dreams of medical school into reality. Being accepted to the University of Arkansas College of Medicine was a turning point in her life. She entered medical school in 1956 and received all of her training at Arkansas Children's Hospital except for a year at the University of Minnesota School of Medicine, where she had won a pediatric internship. Upon completing her internship, she obtained a chief residency in pediatrics back in Little Rock at the University of Arkansas Medical Center.

During her matriculation at the U of A College of Medicine, Joycelyn was the only Black woman in her class. She had to use separate bathrooms and eating facilities. "When I went to medical school," she recalls, "*the Black students couldn't eat in the same dining room with the white students. We had to eat with the housekeeping personnel.*"

Although she did find racial barriers, she was not a woman who was easily discouraged. As a child growing up in a poor family, she had to learn how to survive disappointments, melancholy and despair. Joycelyn has never admitted to any pathological fears about being a person of color.

By the time she entered medical school, she had already suffered most of the insults and invectives that can be inflicted on a Black woman in a segregated society. She dismisses these affronts by saying, "*When you're in medical school, you are so busy surviving, you don't have time to deal with the indignities and discrimination.*"

Because Joycelyn has had to travel a rocky road, she has developed a certain tough exterior that intensifies when she is pushed. When, for example, groups try to confine her in some way or distort what she says, and she senses that racism is the real culprit, she strikes back. While she doesn't talk much about the subjects, Joycelyn bristles at race and sex discrimination. Perhaps that "don't tangle with me" look, which becomes apparent when she senses racism and sexism still loose in her space, is a pent-up reaction to the life of segregation and discrimination she has tolerated for too long.

Reflecting on her medical school experiences in general, Joycelyn has high praise for most of her instructors. Of course, she recalls a few minor disagreements that were not necessarily racially motivated. She also remembers that of those who started medical school with her, she was the only female of the group to graduate.

"Bloom Where You Are Planted"

In medical school, Joycelyn found her life-long philosophy: "Bloom where you are planted." Medical school was also the beginning of her life's work with children. Upon completing a fellowship in biochemistry, she joined the faculty of the University of Arkansas College of Medicine's Endocrine Division in 1964. She became a Board Certified Pediatrician Endocrinologist, the only one of color in Arkansas. Superb in her work, she has developed for the medical school a nationally recognized research and clinical program in the field. She has made many contributions in both basic and clinical research of diabetes and metabolic diseases. She has been recognized with membership on national advisory committees, membership in professional societies and study groups of the National Institutes of Health.

Joycelyn has doctored more than ten thousand babies during her thirty years as teacher and medical doctor. She has taught most of the doctors who now practice medicine in the state of Arkansas. Additionally, she has authored or co-authored some 150 published articles, books and clinical research papers and reports. More importantly, she is recognized as a humanitarian as well. Traveling across Arkansas, one comes into contact with countless parents who will testify that Dr. Elders saved the life of their son or daughter. This work is really what keeps her going.

Working in a profession that has long been dominated by white males, Joycelyn often says that she never felt being Black was a handicap to her. Some Black people are quick to differ with her view and/or misunderstand what she is really saying. She doesn't see the color of one's skin as a problem or handicap unless he or she allows it. Joycelyn's heart has always pained at the thought of injustice. Her life has been spent in the fight against it. She has always tried her best to fight it in a dignified manner. She has never taken injustice lightly or lying down. She believes that being a good example for young people is one of the best antidotes to bigotry.

Never Give Up

I have been with my sister on many of her speaking engagements. She often concludes with the words, "*I may give out, but I'll never give up.*" I asked her on one occasion, "Joycelyn, why do you push yourself so hard?" She quietly but emphatically replied, "*Because I feel that I have something to say, and I will not rest until I have said it.*"

It seems to me, as a minister, that the Word falls on so many deaf ears these days. My sister is refreshing for my faith and hope in the spoken word. When I hear her speak with such power and conviction, I understand why some of my colleagues in the ministry find delight in saying to me, "She should have been the preacher in the family." Her romance with words intrigues even me.

Joycelyn's years of hardship, together with the discipline of medical school, have made her a better person. She often says, "*Everything that I have been through, I really appreciate.*" She has been through a lot. In one way or another, she has lived on the front lines of one battle or another for most of her life. She lives by the Bible verse, Philippians 4:13, "My God will supply all" (KJV).

As unlikely as it may seem, Joycelyn Elders is a real person who has lived a real life. In spite of the many honors, awards, achievements, etc., she has remained quiet and unaffected by it all, just as she was growing up on the farm. She shares the credit for much of her success with her family and close friends. She still enjoys going back to the farm and visiting with our parents, eating country food and baking tea cakes with our mother. She attributes much of her success to the way in which she was reared by Curtis and Haller Jones. "*I felt that my parents really always taught us to do the very best we can, to always be honest, to always help people... I feel that it's something that has to be instilled very early. I feel that the kind of person we're going to be – our hope, will and drive – has really been determined by the time we're 5 years old. So, obviously, my mom and dad did that*" (Russell 25). She cherishes the family codes and the foundation that our parents established for the family. These roots have sustained her.

Chapter Nine

WORK ETHIC AND ROLE MODEL

Hard Worker

Dr. Elders inherited her hard work ethic from our mother and father. She has never forgotten her roots. Dr. Elders still feels at home with her shoes off working in her garden, painting and repairing old houses, cutting the grass on her large John Deere tractor with the bush hog, or doing her routine domestic work of cooking, canning and house cleaning.

She has always worked hard; she has told her two sons many stories about growing up as the oldest child in a sharecropping family of ten. Her son Eric remembers a story about the time she was out working in the cotton field with the whole family. The sun was blazing, the air was hot, but, as usual, being the oldest child, Minnie was determined to set an example for her younger brothers and sisters. She committed herself to picking more cotton that day than she had ever picked before. Inch by inch, row by row, she drove herself, her back stooped over, her fingers stabbing at the prickly bolls; she picked through the heat, through the sweat, through the aching and dizziness and nausea, until she passed out from exhaustion.

Dr. Elders is determined to set an example not only for her brothers and sisters but for everyone she meets. She will not rest; she will not pace herself. I remember once getting a call from her secretary at the Arkansas Department of Health, saying I needed to take her some medicine because she was at home sick. When I went by to see her, she had been running and worked herself down to the point of total exhaustion. She approaches whatever she does with the single-minded passion of the workaholic. She does not believe in wasting time. There is never a moment to lose, whether she is working on a research project or bouncing around cutting grass on her tractor.

Although Dr. Elders has been off the farm for over forty-five years, she still works the hours of the field hand. She starts her day every morning about 3:30 and works until after sunset. She very seldom takes a vacation or time off. I will never work as hard as my sister, but I know it was hard work that got her to the position of United States Surgeon General. She never thinks of her hard work, or her childhood in the midst of relentless poverty as a handicap. She will just say that in our family's tiny shack "*there was no indoor plumbing, no electricity and no self-pity.*" Dr. Elders and I grew up being taught that people should go about their given work without spending time worrying about the "whys," "if onlys," or other theoretical questions one can ask about their life, because, to quote Voltaire, "*work keeps at bay three great evils: boredom, vice and poverty*" (300).

Growing up poor instilled in Dr. Elders a strong desire to work hard and always to do her best. Because of this desire, and in spite of her missing many days of school to work in the fields, she managed to keep up with her school work and graduate from high school at age 15. With the help of a group of Methodist women and a scholarship to Philander Smith College, she was able to study hard and work her way through college in three years. My mother often refers to Dr. Elders as her "little slave girl," referring in part to the fact that, in order to get through college, her oldest daughter had to support herself by staying with a family and doing the cooking, cleaning and other household chores. Dr. Elders was fortunate that because of her childhood situation she learned to cook at an early age. She has always been so preoccupied with work and studying that she has never had time to develop any significant recreational or social life.

Dr. Elders has worked hard with her sons and husband to buy and renovate property. Renovating houses and getting them ready for occupation is not easy work. I have watched her go out to rental property, after working all day at the hospital, and work five or six hours more. I went out a few times to help, but I could never keep up with her; I often wonder where she gets her energy. No matter how hard the job, Dr. Elders' thinking is, "*Never say it can't be done, and don't take no for an answer.*" Her philosophy about life and work is always "to make it happen."

This wisdom has taken her a long way from her home in rural Arkansas, but even today she enjoys going back to the farm to visit with our mother and father. Many of us might have become vain in the midst of the honors she has won, but she has remained the same devout mother, humble housewife and hard-working daughter of a proud tenant-farming family.

Role Model

When my sister came home from the Army for the first time, wearing her uniform and driving a car, she became my role model. I wanted to be just like her. I desperately needed a role model at that time in my life.

When I was growing up on the farm in Southwest Arkansas, I thought many times about giving up and dropping out of school. Many young men and women did just that, largely because of the months of school missed while picking cotton. When I was in the tenth grade, it was a real temptation for me to quit school, run away from home, and try my luck working in the cotton fields or trying to get a job in the sawmill.

My older brother had done this. He had just walked out of the field one day when he had a disagreement with my father about having to chop cotton on Saturday during a ball game. When we got home from the field, we discovered that he had come home, packed a few things and left without telling any of us where he had gone.

About a week later, my aunt in Kansas City wrote and told my parents that my brother was there with her. It was a really emotional time for me, because I really admired this brother and wanted to be like him. It took me about six months to get the notion out of my head that I could run away from home, too. I thought and dreamed for days on end about how I would wait and plan and make my getaway. But it is at least partly true that "time heals all wounds," and after some months I came to myself, realizing that it would be morally wrong to leave my mother, two younger sisters and a baby brother alone to help my father with all the work on the farm. I was only in the seventh grade at the time, but I was a hard worker and by that time could pick over two hundred pounds of cotton a day and do anything in the field that a man could do.

It was during that same summer that my sister came home from the Army on furlough. I knew she had left our farm with nothing but a bus ticket and the address of a college, and now she had a new car and a commission in the United States Army!

She inspired me with a new dream: to finish school and join the Army. I saw military service as a way out, a way of getting off the farm. I wanted to be just like Joycelyn. I went out and sat in her car and started to dream about joining the Army and coming home in my uniform. From that day forward, working in the field was fun. I had developed in my mind a way to transform the present situation and live vicariously in the future. Many times when we were in the field, I would work hard enough to get ahead of the others, so I could be alone dreaming about being in the Army and off the farm. After finishing high school, my dream came true, and I spent three years in the Army, 82nd Airborne stationed at Fort Bragg, North Carolina, as a paratrooper jumping out of airplanes, mostly C-130 cargo planes.

The Army was a good experience for me. I believe it would be good for the country if all young men after high school had to spend at least six months in some form of military service. The basic training makes you want to quit and go back home. But in all of life, in order to reach our dreams, we must surrender ourselves to the steps in the process. For me, the first step was to make joining the Army my first priority. I have learned from Dr. Elders that we can become whatever we dream about and put first in our lives.

The next step is to visualize and make that first priority the dominant desire of our lives. After meeting Dr. Edith Irby Jones while a college student, Joycelyn made it her goal and first priority to become a medical doctor. She wanted to be just like her, and the inspiration of this role model enabled Joycelyn to make that goal her highest aspiration.

Then the process calls for testing our goals and desires out in the marketplace. For Joycelyn, it meant volunteering for the Army in order to have the support of the G.I. Bill to go through medical school. Dr. Elders has a saying that "*whatever one can visualize, conceptualize and actualize can become a reality — with a little motivation, inspiration and perspiration.*"

Joycelyn and I had different motivations for joining the Army. She wanted to get through medical school; I wanted to get off the farm. But the Army was a good experience for both of us. She used her G.I. Bill to go through medical school; I used my G.I. Bill to go through college. Now I am convinced that what Dr. Elders has done for me, and all the rest of our family, is to teach us to believe that we can only reach our dreams through conviction and hard work and studying, not by wishful thinking and following the advice of star-gazers. Just as those who would join the Army must complete their basic training, which calls for hard work and study, those who are successful in life must have dreams and see visions, and they must have a strong desire and a good plan to bring those dreams and visions to reality. For the soldier, it means total surrender to the military authority. For the doctor, it means total surrender to the practice of medicine.

It is natural for everyone to want success. To win success, however, requires labor and perseverance. Dr. Elders' life can serve as a role model, not only for her family, but for people of all ages and races. Dr. Elders can be an example to follow for anyone who will accept trouble and disappointment without giving up—no matter how many times they may give out.

Chapter Ten

ANCHORED BY FAITH

Train up a child in the way he should go: and when he is old, he will not depart from it.
Proverbs 22:6 (KJV)

The Faith that Anchors

It is true that Joycelyn's faith in the Lord is very important to her. She said it herself during the Senate confirmation hearings. She believes that one's faith is a very personal and private thing; thus, she has treated it as such in her life. She is not a fanatic who feeds on emotionalism, self-righteousness and publicity when it comes to her religion. Needless to say, Dr. Elders' approach is out-of-sink with that of the so-called religious right-wing groups who have been so brutally critical and judgmental of her.

Having grown up with Joycelyn, and being her brother, former pastor, confidant and friend, I had the best opportunity, next to her husband and sons, to gain the greatest insight into the faith she possesses. I also know the roots of that faith, as I share those same roots. I would like to share with her critics and admirers my first-hand knowledge concerning the faith that anchors Dr. Joycelyn Elders.

First of all, it is important to say emphatically when it comes to her faith in the Lord, Joycelyn Elders does not need to be defended by anyone. Therefore, let me make it perfectly clear that I am not here intending in any way to defend Dr. Elders and her belief in the Lord. She doesn't need a defender. It is, however, my intent to share concerning the influence I think the teaching of faith by our parents and the church has exerted on Dr. Elders and me.

The Influence of the Church

Our family will never be able to repay the Church universal for the influence and role it has played in shaping our spiritual values and beliefs. Our parents have always been a part of the body of Christ represented by the Christian Methodist Episcopal (CME) Church. Our mother continues to be one of the four active families in regular attendance at the Tabernacle CME Church, the small rural black church we grew up in located in Schaal. Our father has been bedfast for the last five years and is no longer able to attend church. The attendance at Tabernacle is down from what it was during our growing up years, just a handful of members remain. However, these faithful few are determined to keep the light from the lighthouse burning in their community. With great sacrifice, these few recently built a new church building. They sold many chicken dinners and asked for donations from family members and friends to build the new structure which is located on Rural Route One in Mineral Springs.

This location for the new church building makes for an ironic situation, in my opinion. You see, in 1993, the handful of members voted to relocate the church, to no longer be the "little brown church in the wildwood," (or should I say backwoods). The move placed the church in a more visible spot in the community, and nearer the main little road that runs through Schaal. Also the new church is now located on the site where Mr. Will Jones lived, known affectionately as the "Ole' Will Jones' Place." In fact, the church is built on the exact spot where Mr. Will Jones' house and store were located. Will Jones was at one time one of the largest land-owners in Howard County. Along with many other black families back then, our parents also worked the Will Jones' land as sharecroppers of cotton for many years. Now I think it is ironic that through these few people, God, who is the supreme land-owner in the world, seems to be somehow saying as is recorded in Leviticus 25:23, *"the land shall not be sold for ever: for the land is mine; for ye are strangers and sojourners with me..."* (KJV). It seems God has invoked His divine ownership by selecting for His church the very spot controlled by the one-time largest land-owner in Howard County, and the spot on which he allegedly committed suicide in the early 1950's.

I visited the new church during my visit home at Easter, 1995. While visiting, I reminded our Mother of the ironic connection. She, Uncle Bud and other elderly members of the church seemingly had not thought about it. While discussing the subject our nephew, George Watson, came up to me and said, *"Unc, you mean to say that the man who Momma* (our sister Beryl who lives in Detroit) *and all of ya'll used to work for to make your living owned this spot?"* I replied, "Yes!" He said, with a look of surprise, *"man, God is something else, isn't He?"*

As George walked on, he left me filled with the thought that there is something (for lack of a better descriptive term) revolutionary about the Gospel of Jesus Christ. For us to really take His teachings seriously, means to believe that all things are possible. The message to us, though, may be that we are not to reflect so much on trying to figure out what those possibilities are, as much as we are to reflect on what the Lord requires of us. The real lesson from this line of thought is that the Lord does not always demand worldly success of us as disciples. But surely the Lord does require us to be faithful. Nephew George had provided food for a future message and didn't know it.

In that little old country church back home, we learned that the church was indeed a place where you could go and sense the presence of the living God. It was not unusual during worship services for us to experience spiritual awakening and guidance to carry us on through the next week.

The preacher helped us on Sunday to encounter God's love through Jesus Christ, and to experience a new joy and purpose for living. When we were growing up we looked forward to church each Sunday where we could experience that divine love and gain the spiritual confidence that enabled us to go on and live a full and satisfying Christian life despite the odds of the unjust surroundings. In that little, rural church I personally experienced a life-changing relationship with Jesus Christ.

The church was the community and religious family that provided and surrounded us with caring and friendly support which we as young people needed to make it in this old life. The church was our home away from home. It provided many vital blessings to our family, for example, during the time when Momma was so sick the church was there for us. During that time, the church members would bring food and pray that God would restore Momma to good health. Momma saw the church, not as an end in itself, but, as an instrument of the body of Christ to be used especially for sharing with and helping others to find the way.

Within the black community the church was somewhat of a "nation within a nation." It worked to help the little nation within work to free a whole race of people. Yet, ironically, we know that for the most part, the church retains one of the most repugnant vestiges of segregation in our society. I am speaking of the so-called people of God, who say we are worshipping and serving the same God, and who say that they believe that God created us all in His image and that God is love, and yet, we allow the church to be so segregated. Sometime I have to wonder who it is that many people really serve?

As a boy in the late 1940's, I guess I may have experienced my first real consciousness of what a preacher meant to the life of a community of faith. This would have been about the time our parents moved back to Schaal from their stint as war-time workers in California during World War II. During that time it seemed that black ministers would often highlight the issues of the day while delivering their messages. I can remember that one such minister who made an everlasting impression on me was the late Reverend Frisk Walton, former pastor of Tabernacle CME. He had a statement that he read in one of his sermons which was very similar to the passage from Ecclesiastes which reads, "to everything there is a time..." (3:1-4). It went something like:

There comes a time when people get tired:
Tired of being called a boy when you are a full-grown man,
Tired of laughing to keep from crying,
Tired of being kicked around,
Tired of being humiliated,
Tired of being mistreated,
Tired of being segregated,
Tired of living under the threat of death,
Tired of being called everything but a child of God,
Yes! Yes! There comes a time...

As a youngster, Rev. Walton's statement made an indescribable impression on me. I have never forgotten it. It helped me to understand that the church has many roles: one of which is to speak out against injustices against people wherever they are found, yet trying all the while to help find Christ-like resolution to the problems. It seems that sometimes today the church as we know it is impotent to save the world we experience today. The new century which will begin five years from this writing poses us with the question of whether we are ready to face the challenges of the time.

As I look back, I realize that our family owes a great debt

to the church for the role it has played in shaping our beliefs and values. It gave us the strength and courage we needed to face the difficult times then. I pray that it will continue to give us the strength and courage we need to face whatever times are ahead.

Momma's Family Values: Blessed are We with Such a Mother

As I reflect on memories of our time growing up, while I have similar memories of Daddy, I realize that we owe a special tribute to our mother, Haller. Sometimes I am amazed at the wisdom that she possesses, especially in view of the very limited formal education that she was able to obtain. Of course, now, as a grown man, I do understand that Momma's wisdom is largely based in her faith and her understanding of God's word.

Momma was one to practice what she preached. I can remember her teaching us about the need to develop a strong and unshakable faith in God. This was probably the greatest value, or belief, that she held and instilled in us. One may wonder what faith is exactly. In the New Testament Epistle of Hebrews the writer says that *"faith is the substance of things hoped for, the evidence of things not seen"* (Hebrews 11:1 KJV). In verse six of the same chapter the writer continues, *"but without faith it is impossible to please him: for he that cometh to God must believe that he is, and that he is a rewarder of them that diligently seek him"* (Hebrews 11:6 KJV). Momma understood these things about faith and what was required and she insisted that we, too, understood and adhered to it.

Momma Taught Us to Pray

In Paul's letter to the Thessalonians we are told that we should, *"pray without ceasing. In everything give thanks: for this is the will of God in Christ Jesus concerning you"*

(I Thessalonians 5:17-18). Momma understood this scripture, too. She taught us to pray.

What oxygen is to the lungs, prayer is for the meaning of human life. The well-being of the family depends on many things, but in the Jones family, prayer was the greatest of these things. Momma still believes and admonishes us that "the family that prays together, stays together."

In teaching us as children, as soon as we could talk, Momma taught us the most traditional bedside prayer that is still used in many Christian homes today to teach children about prayer. Back then I was a slow learner and it took both Momma and Joycelyn to teach me the prayer. I did finally learn it, though, and I still consider it to be the greatest prayer I know, with the exception of the Lord's Prayer. So, as I stated above, Momma is one to practice what she preaches; therefore, when she taught us how to pray, she would kneel at the bedside with us and teach us the familiar little prayer:

Now I lay me down to sleep,
I pray the Lord my soul to keep.
If I should die before I wake
I pray the Lord my soul to take.

I am now over fifty years old, have been to seminary, and I still consider this one of the best prayers a mother can teach her children. I am glad Momma taught it to us, there is something rich in being blessed with such a mother. You see, at times I still have very vivid memories of my childhood, down on my knees being taught by Momma how to pray.

You might ask why prayer is so important. Paul told us in his writings, but too few of us share that message with young people. Prayer is to life what extract is to a cake. What would a cake taste like without any extract to flavor it? I once made a cake without adding the extract, or flavoring, called for in the recipe. Needless to say, the cake had no taste. That ended my cake baking days. Likewise, when one does not include prayer, as an extract, in his or her life, there is no communion with God to flavor that life.

By the time that I was four years old, Momma had taught me to pray the Lord's Prayer. I see a parallel between what Jesus taught the disciples about how to pray and what our parents taught us. Like Jesus, our parents knew that they would not always be with us. Therefore, they did their best to prepare us for that reality and to instill something lasting in us that would sustain us through the good times and the lonesome valleys of life.

Dr. Elders had this teaching to fall back on during the difficult days of her career. I am convinced that she would not have survived what she faced as Surgeon General and remained sane thereafter if she had not had the benefit of Momma's teaching that prayer does change things. I know she went through some of the darkest nights of her life during that time. I am told that at the darkest part of night only God can help us to see clearly. She would call me long after midnight many nights with questions for which I really had no answers. When I did not have the answers, I'd always refer her to Momma for prayer and counseling. I knew that after she had spoken with Momma, she would feel better.

However, to this day, Momma does not attempt to give us answers to our questions. She knows that when one has certain questions and faces certain problems, she or he really needs the presence of God more than answers to "why" questions. Her usual manner is just to share with us concerning ways of finding solutions to our problems. Of course, her solution to every question and problem in life is centered around prayer and love.

A Mother's Theology

Today I find that many are dwelling in doubt and despair when they could be flourishing in faith. Momma's theology, if you will, centers around teaching her children about a faith which causes one to flourish, no matter what obstacles one may encounter.

Growing up in rural Southwest Arkansas was really hard. In order just to survive, stay motivated and hopeful for a better future, one needed a strong faith in God. We grew up in a Christian home where our theology (our *logos* about *theos* — word about God) was shaped by Momma and our paternal grandmother. In fact, my first awareness of sound as a child is of Momma singing "Jesus Loves Me" to me. Early on the words of this familiar song taught me everything that I need to know about the love of Jesus. I have now been blessed to pass the half century mark, and, because of this song, I have never had any doubt about Jesus Christ as "the way, the truth and the life" (John 14:6 KJV). The Bible for me has always been the authentic Word of God. I did not learn this in any school, I grasped this message from Momma's theology.

Over the years we have learned to cling to Momma's message and we learned to practice what we had learned. Therefore, today, Dr. Elders and I both better understand the power of God's message and command to the community of faith. The Bible teaches us to *"train up a child in the way he should go, and when he is old he will not depart from it"* (Proverbs 22:6 KJV). Jesus also commands us to receive children: *"suffer the little children to come unto me"* (Mark 10:14 KJV). His words, as recorded in the Gospel of John, when he appeared to the disciples after the resurrection were, *"feed my lambs"* (John 21:15 KJV). The point being that what we learn as children is vital; it shapes our whole lives to a large extent. By the time I was ten years of age I knew 90% of all I could ever know about the essentials of the Christian faith. This is one of the major reasons why it is so very important for our nation to re-focus our attention on our children and teaching faith and morals at home. My siblings and I will never be able to repay our parents and the church for the attention and guidance we received from them as children. Our parents gave us something to live for, the church gave us something to work for, and God gave us something to hope for. As the old hymn says, our "hope is built on nothing less!" This faith and hope has seen us all through the difficult days of our lives, especially Joycelyn through her ordeal as Surgeon General.

Momma Taught Us to Say Grace before Meals

As children we were taught to "bless" the food before eating it. I cannot remember a time during my father's active years when he did not say grace before the meal. It didn't matter whether we were sitting around the kitchen table, or were eating from a dinner pail under a tree in the field, Momma always indicated to Daddy to say grace before we ate. Our father's blessing prayer was always:

Blessed Lord, we thank you for the food that we are about to receive for the nourishment of our bodies, for Christ's sake, we pray. Amen.

Back then, the mealtime was used for more than just eating. *"...It is written, man shall not live by bread alone, but by every word that proceedeth out of the mouth of the Lord"* (Matthew 4:4 KJV). It was a time for family sharing and counseling for the children concerning misbehavior which may have been reported to Momma regarding our conduct at church, school, or in the community. Oftentimes, while at the table, the family would also share stories. My father always took his seat at the head of the table and we each had a place at the table. As I think back now, I realize that it was around the dinner table that we were able to learn what it meant to be a family. When one of us spoke, the others listened. I can still remember so well the many meals we shared as a family around the table. I ask myself now, what has happened to that part of family life?

Momma Taught us to Share with Others

We may not necessarily be called to share in the slums of the inner cities all the time, but we are all called to share with others somewhere. Momma believed that God gives us health and strength so that we can share with others the fruits of our labor. Her Christian philosophy in life is, if God could not get His blessing through an individual, He would just stop sending blessings. In Momma's opinion, God has called everyone to share with one another.

Really, sharing with others is nearer the heart of Christianity than being served by others. A Christian is one who serves. Jesus said, *"...who is greater, the one who is at the table or the one who serves? Is it not the one at the table? But I am among you as one who serves"* (Luke 22:27 RSV). We are all called to share in the ministry of Jesus Christ, the ministry of service. We are not called to be self-centered or selfish. Such persons are unhappy persons. They do what they like, but then are unhappy with what they do. Jesus summed it up quite aptly, *"For those who want to save their life will lose it, and those who lose their life for my sake and for the sake of the gospel will save it. For what will it profit them to gain the whole world and forfeit their life?"* (Mark 8:35-36 NRSV). Momma taught us that we would only gain by giving of ourselves to others. Of course, she never promised us that it would be easy, and it isn't always easy. Sometimes we do our very best to share and serve others and are rejected, as Joycelyn was rejected in her role as Surgeon General.

Momma Taught Us to Love Everybody

Jesus taught his disciples that *"no one has greater love than this, to lay down one's life for one's friends"* (John 15:13 NRSV). The most precious gift is the gift of self. On the cross Christ gave himself, his life, for us. The cross shows the length to which God's love will go. The cross has always stood for God's generosity. *"God so loved the world..."* (John 3:16 KJV). The mandate from this is for us to love one another. We are called to respond to the gift of God's love for us by loving in return. Our Momma taught us about love from the time we were born. She loved us and she taught us about God's love for us and she taught us to love each other and everyone around us. Unfortunately it seems that much of our society did not learn this lesson very well. Until we remember and practice this simple truth of loving one another the church will not have much an impact in our world.

Despite our many differences, we are all God's children. We are not to be controlled by anyone or anything except the love of God. Love is the winning quality: it wins when everything else fails. So many young people today are "looking for love in all the wrong places." Everyday I am more and more grateful that in our home, our values were centered on a strong foundation, the foundation of Jesus' love for us and our love for one another. Momma taught us to live by the words of Jesus, *"I give you a new commandment, that you love one another. Just as I have loved you, you also should love one another. By this everyone will know that you are my disciples, if you have love for one another"* (John 13:34-35 NRSV).

Momma Taught Us to Remember the Sabbath Day

As I said earlier, the church and Sunday worship has always been an important part of our family's life. Worship is a celebration of God's victory over death. One of the Ten Commandments exhorts us to *"remember the Sabbath day to keep it holy"* (Exodus 20:8 KJV). This was not only a value in our home, but a rule. To our mother, the Lord's house was the house of prayer and worship, not a house of gossip or play or anything else. Momma taught us that our Redeemer lives, and we learned to worship that Redeemer. We learned very early that there are many things that we might like to play, but worship was not one of them. Worship was devout, reverent and vital to Momma, and through her teaching, to us.

Momma Taught us "Believe in Yourself"

In teaching what we now call "self-esteem," Momma reminded us that we could believe in ourselves because there was always someone bigger and stronger on our side in the midst of life's storms. She would admonish us that, if we lost confidence in ourselves, our enemies could easily overpower us. This is one of the primary values that Joycelyn has relied on all these years, and it has helped her to keep "dancing with the bear." Momma taught us that the only thing worse than losing confidence in ourselves was losing confidence in God. As a result of her teaching we have all held fast to our faith in God and I believe that has allowed us to hold on to our self-confidence in the face of whatever adversity we faced.

As a boy I could never figure out how an ugly caterpillar could become a beautiful butterfly. But always in the summer, my grandmother's flower garden was filled with butterflies. She told me how a caterpillar would spin a cocoon to live in until God was ready to transform it into a butterfly. I never understood the process and I had no use for the ugly caterpillar, but I loved to watch the beautiful butterflies. I think that I learned through watching this process of nature that the power of love is great. We all have choices in life. We can give up when our enemies attack us and spend our lives as ugly old caterpillars, or we can take our experiences and resources, spin them together and fly away as a butterfly. That is what our folks taught us to do. They taught us that we were loved, that we were persons of worth who could take our circumstances and make something beautiful of them.

Momma Taught Us Unconditional Acceptance and Worth

A large part of our learning and developing a healthy self-esteem in our family was the unconditional acceptance we received from our parents and family. The line from an old song says, "you're nobody 'til somebody loves you." We were definitely somebodies, because we knew we were loved. We were always made to feel that we were persons of worth and dignity. This was crucial for us growing up in the time we did when we certainly couldn't have learned this from society. It is likewise crucial today. The deepest need every child has is the need to feel accepted, loved, wanted and appreciated. Deep within the heart of every child or young person is the need to have a parent say to him or her, "well done, I love you, I am proud of you," or words to that effect. Our parents did that for us. Unfortunately, we are not saying it often or loud enough today for all our children and young people to hear and believe.

We have all heard the term "self-fulfilling prophecy." It means that we tend to conform to the image we have of ourselves. We act the way we see ourselves. If we see ourselves as intelligent, we tend to act intelligently. If we see ourselves as bad and unworthy, that is how we will behave. We all need someone to believe in the good in us. This is what our parents did for us. It is what we need to give to our children today. We need to provide for them the acceptance, love, respect and belief in them which they need to be the best they can be.

Jesus never separated people from their worth as a

person or human being. The woman caught in adultery in the eighth chapter of John was not called an adulteress by Jesus; she was not condemned by him. To Jesus she was still a person of value and worth who had simply committed a wrong act. The most difficult part of being a parent is that of separating a child's acts from his or her value as a person. It is one thing to tell a child that he or she has done something bad, but it is another thing entirely to tell him or her that he or she is bad. This is something my parents never did. After chastising me for something I might have done wrong, a few hours later I'd be tugging at Momma's apron and she would reach down and hold me to reassure me that she did not dislike me, but that I was still loved. Not everyone will become parents, but all of us were children at one time. A good parent learns how to separate the child's actions from his or her person and worth. Not to do so leaves eternal scars on the child. We all, then, suffer because of it.

Momma's Most Important Lessons

I have spoken above about some of the important values and beliefs that we shared as a family growing up. These are not the only things we were taught, there were several other important things that Momma taught us:

> Never talk back to adults;
> Eat everything on your plate;
> Never give up;
> Love is always hopeful;
> Forgive others, forgiveness makes love possible;
> Do not say anything bad about anyone;
> Live life by the Ten Commandments;
> "A good name is better than precious ointment"
>   (Ecclesiastes 7:1a RSV)
> Work hard at whatever you do.

Momma believed the saying, "a Christian home is the Master's workshop for character making." Accordingly, she believed that knowing and keeping the Ten Commandments was basic to living a moral Christian life.

Faith in the Face of the Storms

Momma also believed that one major responsibility of parents is to teach children how to weather the storms of life. We can be certain that if we haven't already, we each will have storms to weather in our lives. Momma was determined that we would be able to weather the storms without losing confidence in ourselves, but foremost, without losing confidence in God. She understood that her children would need an anchor in life. That is why she made sure that we understood what it means to have faith in God.

If there is one quality that best characterizes Momma's attitude about life, it is faith. She is a woman of faith. The Bible tells us that without faith, it is impossible to please God (Hebrews 11:6). Faith is the foundation on which the Christian stands.

Momma had such faith. Momma knew, and taught us, that faith was sufficient to see one through the difficult times of life. She believed that storms in life have a way of equalizing experiences and testing one's confidence in self and others. We can be certain, if one has something to hold onto, something to serve as an anchor during life's storms, one should be able to maintain confidence in self and others, including God. Therefore, Momma took seriously her charge to teach us scriptures which would be such an anchor for us in the tough times. She taught us the 23rd Psalm as one such passage. By early grade school, we were expected to know the entire passage by memory. No one failed this test, not even me.

Making our Parents Proud

As our parents prepare to celebrate their 65th wedding anniversary, they can be proud of their work. They did an excellent job of training us "in the way we should go" (Proverbs 22:6 KJV). We are older now, but we have certainly not "departed" from their training.

The guidance that we received is one of the primary reasons Joycelyn has been able to maintain her passion for the possible rather than the impossible. You see, true slavery can exist only when people accept it. Joycelyn rejects it. She understands that life is not without pain, but she knows that there is more to life than pain. The old saying is true for her, "no pain, no gain." She holds on through the tough times and keeps her head up and looking forward to the vision of what she believes can be, just as Momma taught us.

That good ole' guidance of our parents is also one of the reasons Joycelyn has been able to continue her work without uttering unkind words about the President and the White House Chief of Staff, even when many have stated that they believe her dismissal as Surgeon General was baseless. She has also been kind and spoke in favor of the succeeding Surgeon General nominee, Dr. Henry Foster, even though it seems that Dr. Foster succumbed to advice to distance himself from her. Dr. Foster and Dr. Elders attended that same medical school and are good friends. It is rather odd, and unfortunate, that modern day politics can make people reject their friends and love their enemies? Of course, Momma taught us that the Bible said to love our enemies, but Momma taught us that we were never to reject our friends and we were never to say anything bad about anyone. Joycelyn took those lessons to heart and has lived them out in her life.

Strength and Stamina for the Dance

Many people have wondered to me about how my sister keeps on going. I can only tell what I know. There are several things that cause her to stay anchored and give her the strength to keep on "dancing with the bear." The most important are

> The love of God through Jesus Christ
> An anchor of faith and trust in God through Jesus Christ;
> Strong family love and support;
> Fellowship and inspiration of others;
> Faith in the future;
> Belief in herself and what she stands for.

Joycelyn is one of those who has endured many experiences, both negative and positive. She does not expect to be spared the unpleasantness of this life. She does expect that God will be right there beside her as she continues her work and faces the unfortunate experiences of life, like that of her youngest son's drug addiction and the problematic effect it has had on him and on her as his mother. If others can learn from her life, then it will not have been in vain.

There are those who believe that Joycelyn is ahead of her time. On the other hand, there may be those who simply believe she is out of touch. I probably disagree with both schools of thought. I believe she may be trying to awaken us from a deep slumber to what lies ahead of us. I have thought about my sister's work quite a bit; as a theologian, there seem to be several motivating thoughts behind her tenacious manner in which she goes about her work.

First, let me say what many already seem to think. We are on the threshold of the Twenty-first Century, and, somehow, a feeling of unpreparedness looms over us. In many of her speeches Joycelyn has preached about this, she has preached, especially to the Church. I believe she has tried to have us in the Church understand that a crisis lies before us, that the Church, for all the good it does, needs to do more. We must do a better job in the Church of anticipating tomorrow's changes and human needs if we are going to help the people. Otherwise, we may end up like the frog in the kettle, gradually boiled to death. While we can't know all, we need to try harder at anticipating and forecasting and confronting realistically what the future is going to be like.

Second, Joycelyn has often spoken of the need for Churches and other groups and individuals to come together and form coalitions to help solve the health care crises of the nation. She is right in this. There is a dire need for what has been called "servant-leaders" who can discern God's vision for us and articulate it clearly. We need those who will embrace ecumenical leadership and new methodologies to help address the chronic randomness that we fight in the Church, government and at all levels of our society. We need an operational theology with a vision of mission.

Third, if we are earnestly trying to address the kind of crises which Joycelyn has brought to our attention, we must accept the fact that it is time for us to truly be an inclusive society. Not only do we need "servant-leaders," but, more importantly, we need a new generation of "servant-leaders." I am not talking about simply appointing people just to be visible in significant positions. I am talking about appointing and electing those who are willing to set aside their own selfish agendas for one which is truly concerned with meeting the needs of the people. We need a radical new form of "servant-leader" to lead us into the Twenty-first Century. We need a radical new generation of men and women who are from different cultures, races and faith traditions, all committed to working together, cooperatively, guided by the Spirit of God, striving to advance the Kingdom of God in those places where we live.

Jesus Christ gives us a clear example of what a "servant-leader" should be like. He led by giving and sharing power, not by stripping it away from others. He lived and loved the poor; lifted the fallen; washed the feet of his disciples; gave sight to the blind; hearing to the deaf; voice to the dumb; healed broken hearts; gave hope to the hopeless; raised the dead; and, most of all, he gave his life so that we might live. He is our role model, now and for the future. Aren't we called to follow him? Therefore we should be willing to sacrifice our lives, positions, etc. to advance the cause of God's new order of things. Joycelyn Elders sees it this way and has demonstrated her willingness to follow the example.

Fourth, and finally, Joycelyn is an optimist. I am an optimist. We were taught that if we never expect anything, we'll never be disappointed. She and I are optimistic about our future. I believe that if the world was paved with concrete, somewhere, sometime, and somehow, a tiny crack would appear and through it, a rose would bloom. Dr. M. Joycelyn Elders, my sister, is such a rose. She stands as a symbol of optimism and hope, unbeaten by all she has been dealt and still "dancing with the bear" in order to assure us of a better future.

Chapter Eleven

WIND BENEATH HER WINGS

Love and Marriage

Joycelyn graduated from the University of Arkansas Medical School in 1960. In 1959-60 Oliver Elders was basketball coach at Horace Mann High School in Little Rock. (This school later honored Coach Elders by naming the basketball gym after him.) *"Joycelyn and Oliver Elders met when she thumped the knees and checked the pulse of his high school basketball players..., and after a torrid two-month romance, coach and doctor were husband and wife"* (Atkins 65).

Coach and Dr. Elders have many things in common. One of them is that they both enjoy fulfillment in their respective careers. Coach Elders has had a great coaching career in Arkansas. When he retired from Little Rock Hall High School in June of 1993, he was recognized as the winningest high school basketball coach in Arkansas history.

Both Coach and Dr. Elders are great humanitarians. During Coach Elders' career, any of his players could come and talk over their problems with him at any time. Sometimes players who were not able to stay home because of problems with their parents were allowed to come and stay in the Elderses' home until things got better. Coach told me about one occasion on which this happened: "*I went in and told Joycelyn that Tim needed a place to stay, and she just put another plate on the table and never said a word.*"

Early in their marriage they made a vow that there would never be a time that anyone in their family, or friends, would not be welcome to come and stay in their home. I know from personal experience that they have kept this vow. I have had occasions when I needed help as a brother and brother-in-law, and I always had a place to stay and could borrow the money needed to get through a crisis. They took our youngest sister, paid her tuition and let her stay in their home while she attended nursing school in Little Rock. I also remember a time when one of Coach Elders' old basketball players dropped in during the Fourth of July weekend with five carloads of family members—about thirty-five in all. After they had stayed around for a while, Coach asked if they had eaten anything. When they said no, he went out and bought enough food to feed everyone. When the meal was over, he inquired about where they would be staying, since they were passing through from out of town. They said they would try to get hotel rooms in town someplace. Coach Elders said to his wife, "*Shug, fix up places where they can all spend the night.*" She did.

Oliver and Joycelyn have a close and mutually dependent relationship. They help each other work through things. She has said, "*Sometimes we will be up in the middle of the night trying to figure out how to approach certain kinds of problems. I always feel that if I test them out on him and he can't argue me down, then it's a pretty good idea. If the two of us can't figure out a way, then we know it wasn't supposed to be anyway*" (Blount 15).

The Pitter Patter of Little Feet

In 1962, two years after they were married, their first child was born. The child was a boy, and they named him Eric. Having a child meant making adjustments in the Elderses already busy schedule.

In 1964, their second son, Kevin, was born. A third child was stillborn. Several years later, when the boys were both off at college, the Elderses adopted a young patient of Dr. Elders named Nina. The girl was thirteen when she came to live with them and had come from a very troubled background. Despite the nurture the Elderses provided, and all their worry and effort, Nina's life seemed beyond changing. She continued to lead the same sort of troubled life as before and finally moved out from the Elderses' home and was eventually found, along with her boyfriend, shot to death in what is assumed to have been a drug-related crime.

While the boys were growing up the Elderses began to invest in real estate as a small tax shelter. Both parents began to seek information and learn all they could about this specialty. The buying and improving of property turned out to be a good investment for the family and is a business in which they are still involved.

Life during the time that the boys were growing up was congested, and the couple had to squeeze hours into segments in order to have time for each other. Dr. Elders was on call most of the time. In order to spend more time with his wife, Coach Elders visited Dr. Elders at the Medical Center whenever possible. Later, as the boys grew older, he would bed them down for the night and then go visit her. Then there was more time needed to get the boys ready for school the next morning.

Eric and Kevin played the role of helpers to their parents all the way through high school. The parents always involved the boys in everything they did. As they made investments and bought more property, their real estate ventures began to call for a greater commitment of time. Every day after work and school, the whole family would grab a bite to eat and head directly to the newest renovation project and work until dark. The real estate venture eventually took up every hour of their spare time. All summer and vacation time was given to the work of buying and renovating properties, except for some summers when Grandmother Elders would arrange to take the grandchildren on vacation with her to visit relatives.

During these years, Coach Elders took a few summers to attend graduate school and earned a master's degree in health/physical education from the University of Indiana. He made a lasting friendship with Claude Flight, who is now the head of Student Affairs at Virginia State University in Petersburg, Virginia. The work to earn his degree was time consuming, but Coach Elders has many fond memories of his time at the University, especially the time he had to study under Branch McCracken, who was known in basketball as "the father of the fast break."

Chapter Twelve

A CALL FROM THE GOVERNOR

A Noteworthy Career

In 1987, following a distinguished career of almost thirty years as a doctor, teacher, community servant and role model, Arkansas Governor Bill Clinton appointed Dr. Elders to be Director of the Arkansas Department of Health. She was the first black woman to hold that office. Dr. Elders says about her work as Director of the Department of Health:

> *Each of us can do something to help children have an opportunity to develop to their full potential. I always say that when you can move from being a sharecropper's daughter to being the director of a health department for the whole state, you didn't get there by giving up.* (Blount 15)

Indeed, Dr. Elders did not get to this position by giving up, nor did she reach this position and rest on her own laurels. Rather, her work as Director of the Arkansas Department of Health was yet another starting-point for her work to improve the condition of health care, and especially her role as an advocate for children's needs and rights. As Director of the Arkansas Department of Health, Dr. Elders' visions and strategies were for developing a comprehensive plan to address the many social problems impacting health, such as teenage pregnancy, drugs, violence, alcohol, AIDS, homicide and suicide. To assist her in addressing these issues, Dr. Elders recruited the help of schools, churches, civic organizations, local business and community leaders. She was a strong advocate of programs strengthening support for children and reducing unhealthy and risky behavior among youth.

School-Based Health Care

Dr. Elders advocated educating parents in such a way that they would instill in their children a strong sense of self-esteem and age-appropriate health care awareness. In her state position, she came under fire for her support of comprehensive school-based health services which provide primary preventive care for children from kindergarten through twelfth grade. She believed that only through comprehensive health education could the poorest of the poor of Arkansas' children be taught how to take care of themselves. Dr. Elders contended that early childhood education is a cost-effective and preventive measure that reduces the likelihood that such children will end up as dropouts, in prison, or as teen parents. *"It is by all means cheaper to send youth to college than to send them to prison."* The children of Arkansas' poorest parents, Dr. Elders believed, deserved a chance to get a head start on being healthy.

She also believed that both young girls and young boys should be taught to be responsible. She said that *"young men must learn that being a father is more than just donating a sperm."* The school-based clinics offered preventive information to young teenagers, both male and female. But only a very few clinics offered contraceptives on site. The state policy in Arkansas was that the local communities, through their locally elected school boards, had to decide whether they wanted a clinic and what services it would provide. The school boards had absolute control over every decision made by a particular school. Every school board had the freedom to decide what methods it would use to address the problems impacting the social, economic and educational health of its students.

One thing we must keep in mind is that school-based health services, provided through a health nurse at a clinic, work on the same basis as community hospitals. If you are sick and have money to pay, you have the freedom to select the hospital of your choice. Those who are sick and have no means of paying for health services, however, have very little choice other than the city or county hospital supported in part by the taxpayers. School-based health clinics are not for all students. Most of the students in most of the schools in Arkansas are in families whose health services are all provided by a family physician. But there are still a large number of students (in the inner city of Little Rock, for example, or the Delta area of East Arkansas) who are in single-parent or working poor families with no way of paying for health services. Many of these students come from families that help make up the 38 million Americans who have no health insurance.

Dr. Elders understands what it means to grow up in a poor, rural family with no health coverage and to be without the services of a physician. She herself grew up without ever seeing a doctor until her sophomore year in college, and then it was only to hear a medical student making a speech. She never had a physical examination until she enlisted in the Army. She knows that the closest most poor children—black and white—will come to seeing a doctor is a visit from a nurse at school.

Her experience growing up poor in rural Arkansas provided Dr. Elders with a background of personal knowledge about the best means for delivering health services to the families of poor children. To her, the best vehicle for delivery of these services was the comprehensive school-based health clinic. Yet she has been severely criticized by some conservative and right-wing religious groups who seem to believe that one experience fits all: if you are poor and unable to obtain health coverage as a family, it is because you are out of favor with God. This notion is under-girded by the old Protestant ethic that whoever lives right and believes in God will be blessed. Therefore, we should not interfere with God's punishment of the poor by helping them. Another version of this same philosophy was used to prove that God condoned slavery. Now it is being used to twist the words of Jesus, who said that the poor would always be with us: they will, because we, through our irresponsibility, are going to make sure they are. So these groups ride on the backs of poor children by saying that providing health services through comprehensive school-based health clinics is wrong in the sight of God. As a result, many poor children in Arkansas and across the nation are facing a health care crisis because some religious groups promote a religion based upon a God of judgment and not a God of grace and love. And this judgmental God has made them the only messengers of divine truth on earth.

Director of Health Department

The list of Dr. Elders' accomplishments as Director of the Arkansas Department of Health is an impressive one. It includes such things as: helping to locate physicians in rural areas where access to health care had been limited; HIV testing, education and prevention programs; cancer prevention programs; WIC (Women, Infants and Children) formula rebate program; scholarship programs for needy high school graduates; declining teen pregnancy rates among 15-19 year olds; declining abortion rates for same age group; screening program for sickle cell anemia. She worked hard and without fail to improve conditions for Arkansans of all walks of life. She is truly a dedicated public servant. It is such accomplishments, and her commitment as a public servant that is captured in Senator Dale Bumpers speech on Dr. Elders' behalf during debate on her Confirmation as Surgeon General

...I have known Joycelyn Elders on a very personal basis

for a long time. I want to reassure every Member of the U.S. Senate with a personal guarantee: She does not have one bigoted bone in her body. Everybody in Arkansas from the now-President of the United States down to the lowest employee of the Arkansas Public Health Department will tell you that she has been one of the most aggressive and finest public-spirited public servants ever to serve in any capacity in our State. (U.S. Cong. Joint Committee on Printing S11007)

Dr. Elders enjoyed her work as Director of the Arkansas Department of Health and pioneered the way for the state to begin to make progress on better health education and care for our children. It was in this position that Dr. Elders made a name for herself as the "lightning rod" who championed the cause of children and health care, unafraid of the criticism and opposition she met with along the way. The themes which she would go on to advocate as Surgeon General are rooted in her work in Arkansas. These themes are rooted in the real, and all too familiar, crises that Dr. Elders saw all around her in Arkansas and which are all too numerous in our nation. Dr. Elders worked hard as Director of the Arkansas Department of Health to make a difference. Again the words of Harry P. Ward, Chancellor of the UAMS College of Medicine, quoted in the introduction best characterize the work of Dr. Elders at the Department of Health. He praised her for "remolding" the Department of Health into one which was proactive, providing new programs through the schools and communities. He recognized the need for addressing the tough issues which Dr. Elders worked so hard to do. As he said, "in many cases, her positions and opinions caused controversy. In all cases, she opened the window. At least we have been debating the right subjects" (Word 2)

Dr. Elders left a legacy at the Department of Health of programs and positions that seek to address the health crises of the state of Arkansas. She took these same programs and positions to Washington with her, and she continues to take them around the country today, advocating for the care of our nation's health, especially for our children. It cannot be denied that while she was Director of the Arkansas Department of Health that she worked tirelessly for the children. Some may still not agree with everything she did or said, but at least she was doing and saying something to try to help.

Chapter Thirteen

A CALL FROM THE PRESIDENT

"President-elect Clinton on Line One"

I remember the late afternoon when my sister called me at the church to tell me she had received a call from President-elect Bill Clinton inviting her to come to the Arkansas Governor's Mansion to meet with his cabinet appointment team. This call came just a few days after he had nominated Dr. Donna Shalala to head the Department of Health and Human Services. I knew that this position was the one for which Joycelyn had considered herself best suited. Contrary to what people may think, Joycelyn did not lobby for any position in Washington. In fact, she enjoyed her position as the head of the Arkansas Health Department so much that she said she would not even consider going to Washington unless she could select her position. Now the position she had selected had been filled, and she thought the President had nothing to offer her which even came close to giving her the satisfaction that she received from her present job.

"Go to Nineveh"

I listened to her as she went on to make her case about what she would have to give up if she left her job at the Health Department: she would have to give up her home, she wasn't sure at that point that her husband wanted to go, etc. Since her mind was already made up, she saw no need to go over to the Governor's Mansion to waste Mr. Clinton's time discussing an appointment in Washington.

I spent about thirty minutes listening and praying about what I could say to her that would get her to change her mind. I knew her well enough to know that my rational argument would not be able to persuade her. So I used a divine command that had always worked well for the case of the Kingdom of God when a church group would call me to ask if I could get my sister to come and speak to them. Joycelyn grew up in the Black church, where she was very much aware of the scripture passage found in Psalm 105:15: "Touch not mine anointed." So I interrupted her excuses and said in a strong voice, "Joycelyn, God wants you to go to Nineveh. And not only does God want you to go, I want you to go!" I felt that Joycelyn was being called to go to Washington just as the ancient Hebrew prophet Jonah had been called to go to Nineveh. I was afraid her job might be equally as difficult, but I knew the Lord was with her.

Joycelyn countered with a comment or two like "If God wants me to go, He should come and tell me Himself."

"He already has," I said.

After dealing with my sister and making my point in this way, I am now more convinced than ever that ministers of the Gospel too infrequently call upon or invoke the words "Thus saith the Lord" when we confront the people who, like the ancient Hebrew prophet Amos, work in the King's chapel under the King's priest Amaziah. Amos had spoken to the people of Israel about their false piety and using their prosperity to oppress others. His was not an easy message to deliver, but, then, a prophet's message rarely is. Amos was not afraid to stand up to the elitist, pietistic attitudes of his time. We must not be afraid to do so today. We need persons who can be the servants of the Lord today, who are not afraid to speak out about what is wrong with our affluent society. When we find those who are being called to do so, we must not be afraid to encourage them. Perhaps we too often minimize the ways that God speaks to us and calls us to service and ministry. I know that my sister's work is ministry — reaching out to serve and help others, to make their lives better. I believe that God calls each of us to some ministry; God calls each of us to help others realize their full potential. I was convinced that God was calling my sister through the President-elect.

We ended our conversation, because the time had come for her appointment with the President-elect, and the rest is history.

Chapter Fourteen

THE CONFIRMATION

<u>Hurry Up and Wait:
The First Scheduled Hearing Date Comes and Goes</u>

The day Coach Elders and I arrived in Washington to be with Dr. Elders during her hearing before the Senate Committee on Labor and Human Resources, as soon as I saw my sister, I knew something was wrong. She said, "hello, how was your trip to Washington?" She then asked, "have you read the paper?" We said, "not really," because we had left Little Rock so early that morning for our trip to Washington that we did not have time to read the morning paper. Dr. Elders then asked her secretary to share a copy of that morning's *Washington Post* with us. The headline read "Hearings on Surgeon General Nominee Postponed." The article recounted accusations against Dr. Elders of unethical financial dealings while serving as a director of the National Bank of Arkansas Board; accusations against Coach Elders for not paying Social Security taxes for a nurse who cared for his ailing ninety-seven year old mother. It also told of an incident when Dr. Elders supported a decision by top Arkansas health officials to withhold information about some possible defects in condoms distributed by the state. The article related opponents' claims that Dr. Elders had been double-dipping because the State of Arkansas was paying her for her time and vacation days while she was being paid by the federal government as a consultant. And the article rehashed all the now familiar issues used to oppose Dr. Elders, her stands on: teenage pregnancy, health education, sex education, condom distribution, abortion rights, etc. All those charges, on the day the confirmation hearing was to begin, and little did we realize they would be just the beginning of the opposition she would face.

After reading the newspaper article, Coach Elders and I went with Dr. Elders to a conference room to meet with some people from the Department of Health and Human Resources to hear about the reaction of the Senate Committee on Labor and Human Resources to the article. In the conference we were told what that the Senate Committee leaders had met and decided to postpone the hearing for one week to allow time for Dr. Elders' opposition on the Committee to build a stronger case against her nomination as Surgeon General. The two Senators leading the opposition were Dan Coats of Indiana and Don Nickles of Oklahoma, with Don Nickles working the hardest of all to discredit Dr. Elders. It irked me to no end to see Senators Nickles and Coats living in their fantasy world where they thought all they had to do was twitch their noses and snap their fingers and disqualify my sister from becoming Surgeon General. It always surprises and saddens me to see people who are on hate-campaigns who claim to be doing it out of their Christian beliefs. Nowhere that I can find does the Bible teach that it is alright to hate and seek to destroy someone in the name of the faith. Dan Coats would go on to question Dr. Elders harshly during the hearings about a statement she made about the "religious non-Christian right." It seemed to me that he was an apt representative for that group. Senators Nickles and Coats seemed to want to enforce their conservative views on the American people and refused to give Dr. Elders an openminded hearing. This is ironic given the statement made by Coats' press secretary in an article in *The Washington Post* on Friday, July 23, 1993. Coats' press secretary said that Coats was particularly troubled by Dr. Elders' outspokenness and that Coats believed that "one of the most important attributes that one brings to bear in the surgeon general's position is the ability to build coalitions and be temperamentally fair-minded" (Schwartz A4). It seemed Senator Coats expected "temperamental fair-mindedness" of Dr. Elders, but he was exempt from it in his position on the Senate Committee. Politics, fairness and open-mindedness often seem to be mutually exclusive terms. Certainly the politics involved in my sister's confirmation as Surgeon General and the time she served seemed to be anything but fair and open-minded. The selfish political posturing of people like Nickles and Coats prevents our country from making progress in the areas in which we so desperately need to make changes.

The Stones They Cast

The charges which delayed the confirmation hearing, leveled by Coats, Nickles and other of Dr. Elders' opponents, initially focused on the two issues reported by the media: Dr. Elders' role on the board of the National Bank of Arkansas and the lack of payment of Social Security taxes by Coach Elders. Dr. Elders' performance with regard to her financial dealings with the North Little Rock Bank Board are a matter of record. She was required to make full disclosure to federal banking officials, and she did that. Yet Senators Nickles and Coats would press this issue in the hearing and Senate debate, even though there was nothing left to disclose. There were never any allegations by federal banking officials of personal wrongdoing on Dr. Elders' part. As a board member, she did not play a significant role in any of the banks' day-to-day operation. The bank was started in 1982 in a very competitive market. In March of 1988 it had undergone a hostile take-over. The founding Board of Directors, of which Dr. Elders had been part, had been removed. The new Board members bought enough shares to gain the hostile controlling interest in the bank. Even the lawyer for the opposition group of board members who made the hostile take-over admitted as much. The investigation into the lawsuit found no evidence of criminal activity on the part of the directors, and the lawsuit was amicably settled to the satisfaction of both parties.

Founded when speculations were high, the bank did good business during the beginning years. Unlike many savings and loan institutions no one lost any money as a result of the hostile takeover, except for the founding directors. The bank is still in operation and doing very well. Dr. Elders, along with other Board members, were cited in a federal report for violating national banking laws relating to their failure to properly supervise bank management. When the issue came up in the hearing Dr. Elders stated, "*I, along with other members of the National Bank of Arkansas, was reprimanded by federal officials for violating national banking laws.*" However, she said, "*investigators found no criminal activity on the part of any board member and I was not the target of any further inquiry.*" The one point that should be made about this whole bank allegation is that no group of business persons would be dumb enough to make a hostile take-over of a bank that was losing money. Senators Nickles and Coats made more out of Joycelyn's bank dealing than they made out of the $10 trillion that the American taxpayers are burdened with over the Savings and Loan fiasco that happened on their watch as Senators. They likewise spent more time on this non-issue than they did asking questions about and seeking ways to work with her on preventing many of the health crises of our country.

As for the charges of non-payment of Social Security taxes, a favorite theme of this out-of-power party during all the confirmation hearings of early Clinton nominees, it was once again a virtual non-issue. The incident in question was payment of Social Security taxes for a nurse who cared for Coach Elders' ailing mother. By this time the back taxes had already been paid, along with all applicable penalties. This incident involved Coach Elders' family and arrangements made originally by his father. Dr. Elders did, certainly, help in caring for Mrs. Elders, who had Alzheimer's and lived in the Elderses' home, but she was not responsible for any legal or financial matters concerning her mother-in-law. However, when, in preparing for confirmation, Dr. Elders learned that the taxes had not been paid, she and Coach Elders took action to see that the matter was rectified. Dr. Elders only fault in this matter was in not knowing everything that her husband did regarding his parents' business dealings—hardly a fault for anyone who wants to stay in good graces with their in-laws. I suppose the other fault in Dr. Elders in this regard is that she cared enough about her in-laws to have them live in her home and work during her hours at home to care for them. Again, hardly a fault when it comes to being a decent, caring, Christian person.

"If It Seems Slow, ...Wait For It" (Habakkuk 2:3b RSV)

The opposition's newly raised charges and resulting postponement of the hearing meant more worries and burdens for Dr. Elders and her family. It meant another week of anxiety and another round-trip airline fare for Coach Elders and me. It meant another week of being subjects for headlines in the newspapers and other media. During the next week there were many groups discussing the pros and cons of Dr. Elders' qualifications for the position of Surgeon General. Many conservative religious groups and right-wing politicians used this delay to dig for information they could use against Dr. Elders and to take to the airwaves and print stating their opposition to her nomination. Today it almost seems that one person with media coverage makes a majority. At the same time, more than five hundred major groups and organizations came out, wrote letters and held news conferences in support of her nomination. This media campaign was a barrage of information and misinformation hurled at the public and at the Senate Committee on Labor and Human Resources. In an attempt to approach the nomination from a bit different perspective, and to give the Senate Committee a family perspective about my sister, I was asked to write a letter to Senator Kennedy. I did so in order to share with them who my sister is from my perspective. In the letter I sought to lift up the points about Dr. Elders that could not be captured in the information and misinformation that was rampant in the media. I wanted the committee to know Dr. Elders as the woman of integrity and ability I knew her to be, one who had come to this point in her life through her own effort and commitment. I summarized her life and work as follows:

> *I consider Dr. Elders to be one of the best role models anywhere. She may even be considered a pioneer. She is known by me as the oldest of eight children born to our sharecropper parents. Until June 20, 1993, I served as Dr. Elders' local minister for the last eight years. She has held within her the conviction that "even the poorest citizens in the United States should have ready access to preventive health care and comprehensive health education." She has held this conviction for as long as I can remember. Likewise, she has fought passionately to give life and meaning to her belief. It has not been easy for her. I am sure that during her confirmation hearing, she is likely to tell you with candor, that she has and still encounters trouble, disappointment and road-blocks, but she plods on. She does not faint or lose sight of her vision.*
>
> *Dr. Elders did not reach the post for which she is to be considered (the summit of her career) in a single bound. She mounted her climb round by round. It may be said that her life epitomizes the "great American dream." This is one reason why I say Dr. Elders' life may be viewed as a role model for anyone – the youth, elderly, whites, blacks, browns, yellows, reds, all of us. She was willing to toil endless nights, beginning at the foot of the hill and working slowly to the top. When she was only four years*

old, she walked five miles a day to catch the school bus. She had to learn how to cook at age five to help take care of seven sisters and brothers while her parents worked the fields. She performed many chores which included pulling corn, stripping cane, sawing wood with a crosscut saw, baled hay, helped our father stretch coon hides for money to buy food, picked and chopped cotton, milked cows, fed and slopped the hogs, made fires in the fireplace and cook stove, picked may drops and peaches, pulled peanuts, dug potatoes, picked cucumbers and dewberries and helped our father clean out the barnyard to fertilize the cotton and corn fields. In addition, she, made it possible for her seven younger brothers and sisters to get off the farm and go to school. This had to be a great sacrifice for her and her husband, Oliver Elders, but she did it anyway. Therefore, when anyone wants to talk to me about family values, I point them to my sister and what she has done to help her parents and siblings to improve their lives.

At the age of 15, Dr. Elders left the farm where our parents were sharecroppers in Schaal, Arkansas, with nothing but a bus ticket and the address of Philander Smith College in Little Rock, Arkansas where she literally scrubbed floors as a maid earning money for her college education. She received her Bachelor of Science Degree at or about age 18. She then joined the U.S. Army, served her enlistment and was honorably discharged. Dr. Elders then returned to Arkansas, earned her Medical Degree in 1960 and later became a staff Pediatrician. Following a distinguished career of almost thirty years as a doctor/teacher, Dr. Elders later earned the distinction of being the first black female to become Director of the Arkansas Department of Health where she serves as she prepares to face the upcoming confirmation hearing.

What I had tried to point out in this portion of the letter was that Dr. Elders had become the person she was, in the place she found herself, because of the hard work and determination she had shown all her life. I wanted to convey to the Committee my belief that her background would stand her in good stead for the tasks she would face as Surgeon General. I went on in the concluding section of the letter to talk about the values that I believe Dr. Elders' embodies, values which were formed throughout our growing up years. I concluded the letter as follows:

Senator Kennedy, I write this letter in strong support of Dr. Elders to you, not because she is my sister. Instead, without qualification, she is an excellent and respected professional in her field. She is also a humanitarian. She cares about people in general, their needs and their welfare in a way that makes her want to help in some way. She is able to use logical thinking, specialized training and concern to work with others to help define and solve problems. Senator, I want you to know that I sincerely believe that when my sister becomes "America's Doctor," if confirmed as the U.S. Surgeon General, the entire nation will have the opportunity to receive the gifts of Dr. Elders, gifts that I have known since I was a child.

In addition, Dr. Elders is a good mother, wife, daughter and a woman who holds and practices firm religious beliefs. As her pastor and brother, unequivocally, she is a person of integrity and good moral character. She is indeed a good role model for those who are willing to make the sacrifices to pay the awesome price that she has paid to achieve her dream. Yes, she sought the mountaintop as her personal goal, but she has never left her public service duties undone. She perseveres for all people, especially those who cannot help themselves — the children. She believes that we must save the children, bring them to their own, if we are to save America and the world.

Senator, once again, it is truly my pleasure to recommend for your consideration, President Clinton's choice to be the U.S. Surgeon General, my big sister, friend, and parishioner, Dr. M. Joycelyn Elders. I firmly believe she will be an asset to our great nation in this office for which she is nominated. As her brother, friend and personal counselor, I ask for your support and prayers as Dr. Elders prepares to take on her new task in Washington, D.C.

Needless to say the letter was a labor of love and one which I hoped would somehow help the Senate Committee to have a more holistic view of Dr. Elders. It is easy to pull statements out of context, to read and hear stories in the media which combine facts and innuendo, and build any case one chooses. It is another thing to be confronted with a whole person, whose very real life experiences have brought her/him to a particular place and time. It was this whole person I hoped the Committee would see and know when Dr. Elders came before them to testify. I was confident that she would be fully herself and speak truthfully and in a straightforward way when she testified, and I hoped that the Committee would keep in mind where she had come from and who she was as they listened. I knew that Dr. Elders had "a long row to hoe" with the hearing and I knew that there would be a lot of issues raised which would be controversial. I trusted Dr. Elders to remain constant in her approach to them, I hoped for an open-minded hearing by the Committee and I was waiting for the things I knew her opponents would throw out.

Fighting Words or Fundamental Ideas?

Many of the issues raised by Dr. Elders' opponents were

pretty much those to be expected, with the following being among the most controversial: condom distribution; prostitution and pregnancy prevention; school-based clinics portrayed as a vehicle to promote abortion; and a pro-choice stand on the abortion issue. These issues were the topic of much of the questioning by the Committee during the hearing and of their speeches during debate on the Senate floor. Dr. Elders' detractors sought to focus the hearing and Senate floor debate on these "hot" topics and, in so doing, to emphasize her outspoken stands and the controversial nature of much of her work. It is important, then, to look at these points of opposition and to understand what the real issues were around these topics.

"Condom Queen"

First there was the issue of condom distribution in state clinics. At issue, in particular, was the Arkansas Health Department's judgment when its board did not inform the public of some faulty condoms dispensed in a few clinics. However, as soon as the Health Department discovered the four defective condoms (out of millions), they reported this information to the proper authority, the Food and Drug Administration. In a meeting called by Dr. Elders' Deputy Director, Tom Butler, who managed the day-to-day activities of the Health Department when Dr. Elders was not in the state, the officials in charge of this area concluded that a public recall would undermine the public's confidence in the use of condoms. When Dr. Elders was briefed about the situation and the action taken by her supervisors and health officials, she supported their decision. Victor Zorana, a spokesman for the Federal Department of Heath and Human Services, defended the Arkansas Department of Heath's decision. He said that the Arkansas Department of Health did the right thing and making it a part of the confirmation process was "a complete non-issue," (Fullerton 18A). Also, as was brought out in the confirmation hearing, the manufacturer of the condoms in question, Ansell, Inc., shipped orders to over twenty other states. Arkansas was the only state to report on the possibility of defective condoms in the distribution process.

Of course, the larger issue surrounding this incident is the distribution of condoms through the state clinics and the advocation of their use. Many have claimed that the distribution of condoms through state clinics would somehow promote sexual activity among our youth. Statistics show, however, that our youth today don't seem to need anyone to promote sexual activity among their age group. The Children's Defense Fund's *Children 1990 A Report Card, Briefing Book, and Action Primer* reports the alarming statistics. According to the report, during only one day in the lives of American children, 2,795 teenagers get pregnant; 1,106 teenagers have abortions; 372 teenagers miscarry; 1,295 teenagers give birth; 7,742 teenagers become sexually active; 623 teenagers get syphilis or gonorrhea (4). What is necessary, unfortunately, is for us to address realistically the problems that already exist, while working to eradicate those problems in the future. Dr. Elders understands this and has sought to do this through the programs she has instituted and advocated which include broader sex education and education about safe sex. We must get rid of the denial game we play with ourselves regarding teen pregnancy. Children having children is an oxymoron. It speaks more to the inappropriateness of our family values than the behavior of our young boys and girls.

This is not an easy, or popular, topic to address. As ministers, teachers, and parents we all teach abstinence and that the only truly safe sex is through abstinence. I agree with an older member of a church I served in Louisville, Kentucky who said on the subject of safe sex, that "no sex is safe sex." This was a dear lady who had retired from her profession and was very mission-oriented in her religion and she was saving herself for Jesus when she got to Heaven. However, while I could not agree with her more, as a pastor, I know that over half of our young teenagers are sexually active. In fact, I just got off the phone a few hours before this writing talking with a young teenager who was pregnant. She is a good person and has been in the church all her life. Yet she made a mistake, a mistake that God's love and grace can cover. A few years ago I knew another young teenager who got pregnant and gave birth to a child. I have never seen a church reach out to anyone with more love and compassion than they did to that young teenage mother. Nevertheless, I witnessed a real sacrifice on the part of many people to overcome their true feelings in order to reach out in love to that young teenage mother and her baby. The family handled it real well, even though it called for a major adjustment in the life of the whole family.

So, the question we must answer is "how do we make 'just say no' plausible?" Our young people who are already sexually active, whether we want to believe it or not, will not "just say no" to early sex unless we provide them with opportunities to say yes to a good education, a good job and a good reason to delay childbearing. A lot of the problem with our teens is not just that they get involved in sex too soon, but we as parents, churches and schools offer too little, too late.

I hope that, at some point, churches, schools and public officials will come together and conduct community-based sex education and abstinence workshops. We must confront the enemy which is us. We must find a way to reach and teach the unwed about unplanned and unwanted children. We have a community problem. It is no longer just a problem of teenage pregnancy. Teen pregnancy is now a nationwide crisis causing a major drain on every aspect of society. The federal government also must work in coalition with local governments to address this crisis. Many of our teenagers are sexually active and are not receiving education or preventive information to assist them in facing the challenge of such high risk behavior. Many parents, teachers, ministers and elected officials still have their heads in the sand and refuse to acknowledge that the rise of teen pregnancies, also now combined with drug-addicted babies, is a crisis. Teen pregnancy is now becoming a criminal problem. Carl T. Rowan, in his book *Breaking Barriers*, writes,

> *You can trace a large measure of the social malaise within America to the fact that federal and state governments are literally forcing the poorest women in the land to deliver babies they do not want — babies brain damaged in wombs, babies whose mental and emotional development is stunted in infancy: children who will become victims of such mind-warping neglect, abuse, exploitation, that their lives will be dominated by hopelessness and rage that provokes criminal outbursts against everything and everyone around them. (351)*

I have gone to the prisons and heard inmates share with us about the hopelessness and rage and abuse that drove them to criminal activities. This is a problem we must address.

Another crisis which could be averted by the use of condoms is the AIDS crisis. This crisis, brought about by the rise in promiscuous sexual activity and illegal drug abuse, is another reason necessitating the distribution and education about the use of condoms. According to the March 1989 edition of *Consumer Reports*,

> *From the Surgeon General on down, public health officials are advocating condoms to halt the spread of AIDS.*

> Explicit advice once reserved for military recruits now appears as public-service ads on TV screens and transit posters in an effort to save lives. ("Can You Rely on Condoms" cover)

This tragic disease has raised our consciousness and has caused us to address a crucial issue which we have long wanted to avoid. It is sad that it has taken such a devastating disease to get our attention. But, as the article in *Consumer Reports* goes on to say,

> In the absence of a vaccine or a cure for AIDS, condoms are the main product available to consumers that allows them to help themselves avoid contracting the disease. Condoms are a product, but no ordinary product. They are used in the most intimate of acts, and some people believe strongly that matters relating to sex should not be the subject of public discussion. That's why condoms were once kept out of sight, under the pharmacist's counter. But with the spread of AIDS, condoms have become the subject of a vast number of public-service messages to consumers. From subway cars to TV screens, condoms are widely promoted as a product that can avert human suffering and save lives. ("Can You Rely on Condoms" 134)

Beyond the public-service ads, there is a need for even broader education concerning the AIDS crisis and how to help alleviate it. Over the last five years, hospitals and the health care system have come under enormous pressure due to a large increase in the number of patients with AIDS. Five years ago I did not personally know anyone with AIDS, except a few people I had read about in the papers. But now, almost every week, I hear about, or come in contact with, persons who have AIDS. Just one week before this writing a person I worked with for over three years died with AIDS. And just prior to this writing the United Methodist Women in the District where I serve as District

Superintendent celebrated the number of quilts and comforters they had made to give to children with AIDS. The country is in an AIDS crisis. Many families are suffering. Many United Methodist Churches are responding to this crisis through a ministry to persons with AIDS. This is a new mission field for the Church. However, there are still many conservative church groups that claim AIDS is a "punishment from God," and the Church should not minister to people that are "being punished by God." There have been some pastors who refused to visit people with AIDS. Other have refused to visit grieving families or hold a service for their loved one who has died of AIDS. Others refuse to pray for the families and friends of persons who have AIDS. Many preachers refuse to minister to persons with AIDS on one hand, and on the other hand quote scriptures from the Bible, such as "always treat others as you would have them to treat you," (Matthew 7:12a NEB), or "Nothing... can separate us from the love of God..." (Romans 8:39 NEB), or perhaps, "And if one member suffers, all suffer," (I Corinthians 12:26 RSV).

Many persons with AIDS are suffering today and feel separated from the Church and mistreated by the people of God. This only points further to the need for widespread sex education, and the need for distribution of and education about the use of condoms.

Dr. Elders has said in many of her speeches that, "*It is absolutely deplorable that it took the emergence of the AIDS epidemic before the word 'condom' could even be mentioned on television.*" She says that "*the threat of adolescent pregnancy and the transmission of other sexually transmitted diseases should have been more than enough to prompt major 'counter-programming' efforts years and years ago.*"

However, even with a teen pregnancy crisis and the AIDS epidemic, many schools still refuse to teach sex education.

The school officials say let the parents do it, when the evidence is clear that many parents do not have the skills and are too embarrassed to talk about sex with their children. Also, most of the parents that I know would prefer that schools teach their children about sex education. However, this may be a cultural and/or racial preference, because when I listen to most white ministers who will openly make reference to sex from the pulpit, they seem to think that the parents should teach the children about sex education. It seems that often black churches, in particular, have done little more than to moralize about sex. Among the black culture it seems that we have opted for "sex-training," in the backseats of cars and the like, rather than sexuality education programs in our churches. The difference between sex education and "sex training" is vast. Sex education is comprehensive in its scope and preventive in its hope. Sex education is about changing attitudes and behavior. It is about teaching self-esteem. It is not only about teaching abstinence, it is about equipping young persons to know how and why abstinence should be a way of life before marriage. Sex education is teaching the principles of self-reliance. It is about teaching, thinking, living and acting in a responsible way. It is about living by the golden rule. Sex education is about taking pride in being a responsible Christian, knowing that your body is the dwelling place of God. "Sex training," on the other hand, is like closing the gate after the horse is out of the barn. It is about waiting until someone is sexually active before they are told about the facts of life. "Sex training" is about changing partners rather than behavior and attitudes. It is about a particular person in a particular relationship engaging in particular behavior. "Sex training" is about fathers telling their sons to "go out and 'score'" while telling their daughters to "keep things in store." All in all, the question is, would you rather have your daughter involved in sex education or sex training? At any rate, I say let the white parents who will, teach their children, but I am convinced that the black community and the black churches must see that our black children are taught to say "no," period, to sex! But if they do not understand that "no, period" means no sex before marriage and they continue to fill their lives with commas instead of practicing "no period" in regards to sex, then they must be taught to protect themselves and the community. The guiding principle for both whites and blacks today, I think, must be to advocate abstinence, but we must also educate about responsibility. Both whites and blacks must be committed to seeing that our children have access to sex education and not "sex training."

The other issue where sexual activity is concerned among black adolescents is one connected with the changes in our socioeconomic position since the time of the Civil War. Through the last 125 years we have taken people out of the fields at a progressing rate, but we have failed to re-educate ourselves about our socioeconomic attitudes. We have ingrained in us the attitude that procreation was necessary for producing more field hands. But as we have emerged from a primarily agrarian culture, this is no longer a necessary attitude for survival. We must begin to re-educate ourselves about our attitudes toward having and rearing children. No longer is it necessary to be a "breeding ground" for field hands. When we can fully incorporate this attitude into our mindset we can hopefully help to reduce the high rate of teenage pregnancy, sexually transmitted disease and the like.

The controversy over the distribution of the faulty condoms at the state clinics, then, served as a catalyst for raising several other related issues. Dr. Elders' role in the incident, and her stand on this and related issues are consistent with the work she has sought to do to reduce teen pregnancy and sexually transmitted diseases. Her testimony on this issue in the hearing consistently called for a focus on what is best for our children and youth. Her work is focused on helping to make sure that our children have the best possible chance at future success. However, many have chosen to misinterpret her message and her work in this area.

"Ye that are without sin..." (John 8:7 KJV)
"Norplants for Prostitutes" and Male Responsibility

Another example of this sort of misinterpretation of Dr. Elders' message and work grew up around the issue of providing "Norplant" birth control implants for prostitutes. Another "hot" topic which is not usually deemed suitable" for discussion, but which was raised by her opponents in an attempt to derail her nomination.

This issue resulted from a response Dr. Elders made to a caller on the CNBC television program, "Talk Alive." Again Senator Nickles would be the chief opponent on this issue, raising questions and objections to the incident during the Committee's hearing and rehashing it on the Senate floor. True to form, a statement was pulled from the context of the conversation in which it originally occurred and was used against Dr. Elders. Admittedly, in and of itself, it is a rather radical statement, but the radical nature of the many crises of our world call for some drastic response to be made and Dr. Elders is not afraid to step out and consider some new and radical measures. The caller to the TV show asked Dr. Elders what she, as Surgeon General, would do about crack-addicted prostitutes who gave birth to crack-addicted babies. She responded that she "would hope that we would provide them with Norplant so they could still use sex, if they must, to buy their drugs," ("Talk Alive").

Dr. Elders' response to the caller was a response on a live program to a loaded question. Personally, I would never try to answer such a loaded question on live public television. Because as long as we, the American public, are programmed to see prostitution as a concern only about poor women in general, and black women in particular, we will continue to view this as a problem of simple morality from the perspective of a racist, male-dominated society. There was no good answer to this question, and, certainly, no easy answer to it. Any answer that did not provide some kind of simple, moral condemnation was not going to be well received by the "powers that be" in society.

We Americans are taught to believe that prostitution is a female problem. We have been taught this by society, schools and even our religious institutions. The biblical paradigm that we have used to support this claim is found in the eighth chapter of the Gospel of John. In this chapter John tells about some Scribes and Pharisees who caught a woman in the very act of adultery and told Jesus that "Moses in the law commanded us that such should be stoned; but what do you say?" (John 8:5 KJV). Well, what could he say? Jesus, knowing the intent of their hearts, threw the question right back at them when they continued pestering him and said: "He that is without sin among you, let him cast a stone at her." (John 8:7 KJV) Jesus did not moralize or uphold some legalism. He did not condemn the woman, and yet, we have used this story to keep the focus on the woman when it comes to issues like prostitution. It is interesting that this story, like our tendency, focuses on the woman who was committing adultery, but conveniently omits any reference to the man. Joycelyn pointed this out to me in one of our Sunday lunches when I had preached on this text. She asked me, "What about the man?" As usual, she put me on the spot. I had to admit that the story did omit any reference to the man involved in the incident, but Joycelyn was right to ask about the man's responsibility. According to ancient laws the man would have been subject to stoning along with the woman. (See Deuteronomy 22:22ff) The man is not brought to Jesus along with the woman. It is probably safe to assume that the crowd gathered there ready to stone the woman was a crowd of men. Jesus' words, "You that are without sin..." did not directly implicate the men, but perhaps it reminded them of the law which required the death of both parties. At any rate, the story is an early example of the lack of male responsibility and the tendency of male-dominated societies to exonerate men while women pay the price.

We must begin to change the way we approach this issue. It is time for us to examine our attitudes concerning responsibility. This issue has serious implications not only in the debate about implants for prostitutes, but also when it comes to the issue of teenage pregnancy. Male responsibility is something which needs reinforcement in our society. Family planning and sex education have traditionally focused on young females. This strategy appears to absolve young males of sexual responsibility. They become little more than "sperm donors" with no responsibility for the lives created. Procreation has been a way sometimes used by young persons to prove themselves. They feel that they are truly women and men when they are able to be sexually active and the ultimate proof of sexual activity is to have a child. Getting a girl pregnant seems to be a real sign of masculinity and feeds the ego of the young man. What we must do is find other ways to help our young persons feel that they are becoming women and men without having to prove themselves by having children before they are ready. We need to give them opportunities for growth and self-expression in other arenas of life. We must realize that our attitudes and the way we treat our young people contributes to this problem. Often we see trouble when we look at our young people, rather than seeing them as human beings with potential. We must realize that our young adults, boys in particular, are not some primitive creatures who cannot control themselves. We must treat them as rational human beings with potential. Before we can get things right we are going to have to see things straight when it comes to relating to our young people as decent and loving children. This is the underlying issue when it comes to teenage pregnancy and the way we treat issues like implants for prostitutes. We must expand and change our attitude concerning the issue of responsibility.

When the issue of implants for prostitutes was raised by Senator Nickles and discussed in the Senate debate on September 7, 1993, I sat for long hours watching them stone my sister. During those hours I witnessed one white, conservative Senator after another ridicule her for making a practical response, as a scientist and doctor, to a caller's question that not one of them had ever tried to address. They had not attempted to address the issue of what our policy will, or should, be on the growing number of crack-addicted babies being born to prostitutes. These merchants of escapism, Senators who maligned and attacked Dr. Elders for addressing the question, have nothing but a do nothing policy on this issue. Dr. Elders in responding to the caller on live television, without any time to address all the multidimensional needs of crack-addicted prostitutes having crack-addicted babies, answered as a concerned health official. Rather than saying nothing, or dancing around questions like a politician, she answered as a doctor that she would provide Norplant to prevent prostitutes from giving birth to crack-addicted, disease stricken babies. When my sister asked me how I would have answered this question, I said "by castrating every male person in the country over the age of fifteen." She said, "Chess, I am serious, I want to know how would you have answered the question?" I said, "Joycelyn, when I get a question like that I usually tell people I need to pray about that for a while."

Norplant, the hormonal contraceptive implant which is almost 100% effective for up to five years, is just one strategy for addressing this issue. Of course, a politician, minister, social worker, or average "Joe Blow Citizen" might have responded in a different way. They would have responded by following the golden rule, "do unto others as you would have them do unto you." (Matthew 7:12 KJV) Only in this case, many would interpret the golden rule to mean, "do nothing as we are doing now about crack addicted prostitutes having crack-addicted babies."

Dr. Elders' statement around the prostitute still being able to use sex, if she must, to buy her drugs is one of the "funky facts of life." We all say we want prostitution and drug addiction ended. But the actions of many Americans say otherwise. We will never address the issue of prostitution in this country until we can teach our young males to curb their appetite for sex. As long as there is a male market for prostitution, it will continue not only to exist, but thrive. Almost everything in our society tells men that we need sex to prove our manhood, that we need it to sell cars, clothes, vacations and magazines. Thus, as long as we refuse to educate our children about one of man's greatest passions, sex, the issues of prostitution, drug addiction, crack-addicted babies, the spread of AIDS and a multiplicity of social and public health problems will continue.

A related question that has been raised is about the incidence of HIV and sexually transmitted disease infection if we only provide prostitutes with Norplant and allow them to continue to use sex to buy drugs. Dr. Elders recognizes that Norplant does not protect one against STD's and supports the use of condoms by prostitutes and those who are sexually active as a means to prevent the spread of HIV and STD's.

Dr. Elders knows that the issues of prostitution, drug addiction, birth of crack-addicted babies, the spread of HIV and other STD's and teenage pregnancy are major public health problems requiring a multiplicity of solutions including public education, drug treatment and the use of condoms. In all of Dr. Elders' efforts to get schools to teach our children about sex, when age appropriate, through a comprehensive plan of health education, she has given school administrators and school boards this warning, *"the methods to achieve this objective must be undertaken sensitively to avoid indirectly encouraging or condoning sexual activity among teens who are not yet sexually active."* This is the theme running through her work, and it is the one, which, when conveniently overlooked, allows her detractors to have a "hey day" with Dr. Elders' words and work.

Reading, 'Riting, 'Rithmetic and Responsible School-based Health Education

A related issue which Dr. Elders' opponents used against her is the school-based clinic. Contrary to assertions made by many conservative politicians and church groups, school-based clinics do not leave parents out, nor do they promote abortion as they contend. Nationally all school-based clinics require some form of parental consent to involve parents in their children's health care and to protect clinics from any potential liability. In Arkansas, Dr. Elders has said in many of her speeches that *"parents determine whether their children may receive services through school clinics and which services they may receive."* This was a policy first instituted by Dr. Elders and was later encoded into state law. No counseling about, nor reference to, abortion is made in school-based clinics operated by the Arkansas Department of Health.

Dr. Elders says that *"school-based clinics are comprehensive health care centers that provide a wide range of health and social services to adolescents at or near where they spend most of their time, in school."* Dr. Elders believes school based clinics are essential in helping adolescents overcome barriers to health care including: (1) general apprehension about discussing health care problems or inability to negotiate the existing health system; (2) inconvenient appointment times; (3) lack of transportation to health care facilities; (4) lack of insurance coverage to pay for health care; and (5) concerns about confidentiality in seeing a health care provider.

Each clinic is unique in its response to local needs and norms. Dr. Elders contends that *"through programs at the clinics, students learn the consequences of early sexual activity. They are also able to learn responsible decision-making, how to resist peer pressure, and the responsibilities of parenthood."* School-based clinics are just one example of preventative medicine to address what is a major problem in today's society — teen pregnancy.

Dr. Elders believes that comprehensive health and family life education should be taught to all children, starting in kindergarten and continuing through high school. Of course, she says that

> *instruction should be appropriate to the child's ability to understand and need to know. After all, the message that our children get from television and videos, older siblings, and even parents do not respect their ages. Therefore, our children need to know about human nutrition and physiology and the risks of substance abuse, tobacco use, alcohol consumption, abuse of prescription medications (more than narcotics alone) and experimentation with substances that may be offered by friends or strangers. In the same way, they need to be armed with knowledge about human reproductive biology and development. The risks of early and unprotected sexual activity are effectively learned in such a context. We must*

do all we can to empower our children with useful facts and resources. (Elders "Comprehensive" 7)

All in all, Dr. Elders believes,

> comprehensive school-based clinics are needed to provide medical care, including family planning services to all teens. Comprehensive school-based clinics are logical partners of comprehensive health and family life education. If children are taught health promotion and primary prevention and health care, there will be demand for such services. Providing them in school makes them nearly universally accessible. ("Comprehensive" 8)

Students who have access to health care know that someone cares about them. They develop healthy self-perceptions, self-esteem, self-identity, a sense of belonging and motivation to prevent early sexual activity and pregnancy.

Despite these facts, opponents have sought various points to contend that school-based clinics were little more than abortion/sex clinics. One of the charges made by opponents is that school-based clinics are too costly. Dr. Elders contends that there is no evidence to support this charge.

For example, she says,

> in Arkansas, the estimated average annual cost of school-based services is $100.00 per student. In contrast, the estimated annual health care cost per person is over $1,300.00. Thus, depending on the number of students involved and the scope or comprehensiveness of the services provided, school-based health services can be expensive. However, such services are also cost-effective in providing early intervention to prevent costly medical treatment down the road. (Elders "Student" 7)

The facts, then, clearly show that Dr. Elders' opponents are wrong in their contention about the cost of school-based clinics. It is simply another case where opponents refuse to see the whole picture of the services provided by the clinic and are searching for anything to try and keep anything that is remotely involved with sex education away from students. In their narrowly focused quest they are failing to look at the need that exists in our society for certain issues to be addressed. Dr. Elders has continually sought to raise our consciousness and call us to look at the difficult issues. This is what draws the fire of her opponents.

Issues focused on by opponents of Dr. Elders, like the opposition to school-based clinics, generally are merely token issues for their larger agenda. The larger agenda of those who oppose school-based clinics is, as stated above, abortion. Another charge raised by opponents to address this issue is that Dr. Elders used her position as Director of the Arkansas Department of Health to promote a pro-abortion agenda. Although Dr. Elders has repeatedly stated that she wants "*to make every child born in American a planned, wanted child.*" Dr. Elders never used her position to promote a pro-abortion position. She has said in almost every speech she has made through the years that she is about preventing unplanned pregnancies, thereby reducing the need for abortions. One of her favorite sayings is, "*I have never known a woman to need an abortion who is not already pregnant.*" Her position is one which takes seriously the crisis of teen pregnancy and which seeks to prevent unwanted pregnancy, that is very different from promoting abortion. She has sought to stop the problem before it reaches the state her opponents are so sure she supports. The programs she advocates would make 'her opponents' charges null, because Dr. Elders works for programs to prevent unwanted pregnancies before the fact, not to terminate them after the fact. To claim that school-based clinics are about promoting abortion is simply not a reasonable claim. The two issues are not related, except for Dr. Elders' opponents.

When it comes to the issue of abortion, it is true that Dr. Elders would take a pro-choice stand; however, this still does not mean a pro-abortion stand. The two are not mutually inclusive. Dr. Elders has believed in and supported the rights of individuals to make choices about their own lives, bodies and health care. I asked her once whether she thought abortion was wrong. Her response was, "yes," and she gave me a litany of wrongs like it. *"We all know that abortion is wrong, just like war is wrong, racism is wrong, Sunday morning being the most segregated hour in America is wrong, murder is wrong, slavery was wrong, breaking our treaties and almost wiping out many tribes of the American Indians was wrong, stealing is wrong, for some people to have too much and some to have too little is wrong."* The question is what to do about these problems and wrongs; what to do to prevent them? So, when it comes to abortion Dr. Elders supports the right for women to choose, while she maintains a strong emphasis on programs which assure the best circumstances for our children and youth. This means that she has opposed the anti-choice groups whose concern is often so narrowly focused that it falls short of being a true concern for the greater good. Another point of opposition to her confirmation as Surgeon General arose from this stand.

"Love Affair with the Fetus" versus Long-term Care for Children

Much was made over Dr. Elders' statement that, *"Anti-choice groups should get over their love affair with the fetus and start supporting children."* Again, a radical statement, but, if viewed from a broader perspective of the greatest good for society, it strikes at the root of one of the crises of our nation. On the surface it may appear to be an inappropriate statement; however, if considered closely, it is a call issued by Dr. Elders for some anti-choice groups to come down from their ivory-tower thinking about teenage pregnancies. Dr. Elders' hope, expressed in this statement, is that every child born in American would be a planned and wanted child. Perhaps this hope of hers can be likened to what Tom Sine calls the "wild hope of God" in a book by that name (Sine). Dr. Elders has a "wild hope" that we can change our society to one that loves and values children, rather than being a society where children often seem to be viewed as disposable commodities. A case in point of our apathetic attitude toward children was the highly publicized senseless murder of the two young boys by their mother in South Carolina. This event causes me to ask, are children now simply disposable when they get in the way of what grown-ups want to do? Admittedly it can be trying at times for young parents who fail to see children as a gift from God, but rather see them as a burden. Of course, this is compounded by the fact that it is often children themselves who give birth to the unwanted children. This tragedy should cause us to seriously consider the attitude we have toward children. It is unimaginable that a parent could simply murder her/his children because she/he is tired of dealing with them, but yet it happens. When we get caught up in discussions about the right-to-life and bringing children into this world we need to remember how they are treated once they arrive and how they are taken out of the world all too often. We need to worry more about our respect for the sanctity of life that is brought into this world and less about our love affair with unborn fetuses.

Another reality that Dr. Elders has heralded is that teenage pregnancy and poverty are inextricably bound together. Teenage pregnancy is a social and educational problem, but it is also very much an economic problem. The problem with teenage pregnancy is related to the fact that our society has given up on the poor. Poor children are at risk from the moment they are born because they are seen as inherently ineducable by some Americans who feel that education is for the privileged few. Dr. Elders feels that it is counterproductive for young girls to continue having unwanted children who are born in poverty and end up abused and grow up to be abusers themselves. This is yet another reason we need to get over our "love affair with the fetus" and look realistically at the socio-economic horrors of teenage pregnancy.

Dr. Elders' criticisms of anti-choice groups are based upon the fact that their movement against abortion is not matched by a support of legislation and policies that would support aid programs for many poor teenage mothers. Anti-choice groups have not played a prominent role in support of any social or government programs or legislation which support poor children. Much of their approach is to push the problems of poor children and their mothers under the rug, ignoring the fact that they will only come back to haunt us as children with major behavioral problems. They want the children to be born, but they don't work as hard to see that they are properly cared for after they are born as they do to see that they get born. Dr. Elders simply feels that anti-choice groups should be willing to work as hard to support entitlements for children as they work to support the right of those children to be born.

Dr. Elders has simply been willing again to step forward and point out that "the emperor is naked." She points out that we cannot simply advocate one position without understanding the ramifications it has in other areas. We have a choice. We can support the anti-choice, pro-life, plan of allowing all children the right to be born and of doing nothing for them after they are born, or we can support Dr. Elders' plan of prevention through sex education. Our choice will determine whether we will be in an even worse social crisis down the road, or whether we will be working to see that all our children have a better chance than we did.

We must work to see that all our children have the rights they are entitled to, which means much more than the right to be born. Many of the children who are allowed to be born in this country lose their rights and have no advocate for their rights. Many are treated as non-citizens. Alarming numbers of children are not immunized, they are poorly educated, poorly housed, poorly fed, and poorly treated. They are exploited, brutalized and denied their rights which some groups claimed to be working so hard to ensure. No one should have the right to sentence a child to AIDS, or crack addiction for life. Yet by not fighting to improve the condition of children born in poverty, we are doing just that. We have given equal rights to everyone in this country except children. Children's advocates are in an ongoing struggle to ensure full citizenship for them. This is what Dr. Elders has fought hard to ensure and why she has spoken out against groups who do not join in this fight.

Anti-choice groups need to be equally as adamant in their stand for children after birth as they are for unborn children. These groups have a half-and-half philosophy. They have a "half-free/half-slave" philosophy. They fight for the "right to life," but do not fight to see that that "life" is ensured of freedom and all the rights connected. Until this half-and-half philosophy is ended, Dr. Elders is right, they only have a love affair with the fetus. This is the truth as I see it. The anti-choice, "pro-life," group, which have an almost exclusively white following, seems to care only about the unborn white fetus. When the same group is polled on matters which are directly related to blacks they oppose affirmative action, public schools and bussing to achieve racial balance. Thus, equal treatment for the black child is nowhere to be found in the anti-choice agenda. Too many poor black children are being born unplanned and growing up unloved and unwanted. One clear indication of this problem is that in America today, even after the passage of the Civil Rights Act of 1964, more black males of college age are in prison or under the control of the criminal justice system than are in college. The anti-choice movement has spent an inordinate amount of time developing plans and strategies to protect the fetus, but hardly any time at all to develop a plan to save the children once they are born, a great many of which are being born to young black women and grow up in poverty. Statistics show that

> *nearly 40% of all black females become mothers before the age of 20; rates of gonorrhea among black adolescents are increasing, while overall rates are declining among other races and age groups. Gonorrhea rates are more than seven times greater for non-white than white 15-19 year old females; black children less than 15 years old represent 15% of the populations, they represent 54% of the AIDS cases reported from 1981-89 (Elders "America's" 6)*

Further statistics show that

> *compared to a white child, a black child is:*
> *almost three times as likely of being born into poverty*
> *two times as likely of being born to a teenage mother*
> *two times as likely of being born to a mother who has no prenatal care*
> *three times as likely of being born at a dangerously low birthweight (less than 3 lbs. 5 oz.)*
> *two times more likely to die in the first year of life*

Compared to a white child, a black child has:

a forty percent greater chance of being born to a mother who did not complete high school
three times the chance of being in an educably mentally retarded class
less than half the chance of being in a gifted and talented class
two and a half times the chance of being suspended from school

Compared to a white child, a black child is:

three times as likely to be living with only his or her mother
four times as likely to be living with neither parent

Compared to:

a white infant, a black infant is seven times as likely to die of HIV infection
her white age peer, a black female age 15-24 is five times as likely to die of HIV infection
his white age peer, a black male age 15-24 is three times as likely to die of HIV infection
his or her white age peer, a black child age 1-4 is three times as likely to die by firearms
his white age peer, a black male age 15-19 is almost four times as likely to die by firearms
his white age peer, a black male age 20-24 is four times as likely to die by firearms. (Elders "Portrait" 1-2)

These are the kinds of issues that Dr. Elders has been trying to address with more hindrance than help from most of the members in the anti-choice movement. They are the kinds of statistics that Dr. Elders sought to address as Surgeon General. It boggles the mind to consider how some could be so upset about a person speaking the truth. There is nothing wrong with having a love affair with the fetus. I think every person should have a loving concern to see that the rights of the unborn are protected and God's laws respected. However, our mission does not stop with just seeing that children are born. We must see that all children are fed, clothed, housed, educated, protected, respected and loved. It is not a loving thing to be concerned only about children being born and not about what they are being born into. Dr. Elders has worked hard to point out that children in our country make up the membership of what she calls the "5-H Club." She says, "*America is the world's wealthiest nation, but today our poorest Americans are the 12 million children who live in poverty. They are members of the 5-H Club – the hungry, the homeless, the helpless, the hugless, and the hopeless.*" Dr. Elders has worked tirelessly to try to reduce the membership in this club, but she has been faced by opposition from groups like the anti-choice groups who would do little to help alleviate the situation. Dr. Elders says,

> *The children, who are our only hope for the future, are hanging by a very slender thread to any hope for their future. Until we address the problems in our society which have resulted in children being poorly housed or homeless, poorly fed, poorly educated and lacking adequate health care, we, as professionals in the field of pediatric care, will be continuing to hand out band-aids when what the patient needs is major surgery. ("Portrait" 2)*

It is "surgery" which Dr. Elders advocates and band-aids proposed by the opposition.

"Anti-Catholic" and Not Good Enough to Boot

Two other issues raised by opponents which merit a brief mention are that Dr. Elders is "anti-Catholic," and the she is simply not qualified professionally to be Surgeon General.

A great deal was made of the "anti-Catholic" charge in the debate on the Senate floor. This charge came from a statement Dr. Elders made about abortion and the stance of the Roman Catholic Church on this issue, "...*look who is fighting the pro-choice movement is a celibate, male-dominated church.*" While this statement is made in very harsh terms, and does not give fair and equal attention to the theological issues behind the stance of the Roman Catholic Church, it cannot be denied that the Roman Catholic Church is a male-dominated institution. Dr. Elders did write letters apologizing for any offense caused by these remarks, but continued to stand by the basic point of the whole statement, which was that women should have the right to make choices concerning their own bodies and their own health care decisions.

As for the other charge, that Dr. Elders was not qualified professionally to be Surgeon General, this claim does not hold water when the facts are reviewed. By professional and life experiences, Dr. Elders is one of the most qualified individuals to ever be nominated as Surgeon General. The details of her life and professional experience as detailed throughout this work show that she is qualified. She has been a nationally recognized leader in pediatric medicine, as an expert in the care of pediatric patients with insulin dependent diabetes; she has published over 150 scientific articles in medical publications; she served very effectively as Director of the Arkansas Health Department; she served on the Executive Committee of the Association of State and Territorial Health Officials and was unanimously voted to the presidency of the Association by her peers; she has doctored more than 10,000 babies; and has taught most of the doctors who are now practicing medicine in Arkansas. A list of some of her accomplishments during her tenure at the Arkansas Department of Health includes:

> 1. Childhood immunization increased by 23%.
> 2. Doubling the Dept. budget to provide 1,000 additional employees ensuring quality health care to even most rural communities.
> 3. New revenues were awarded by federal and private grants.
> 4. More health units developed than during any previous administrator.
> 5. Visits to Public Health units increased by over 250,000 due to increased accessibility.

These facts speak for themselves. They show that Dr. Elders has proven that her commitment is to improving health conditions for all concerned.

In spite of the opposition and charges made against Dr. Elders during the confirmation process, she remained constant in her commitment to improving health care conditions for all, reducing teenage pregnancy and working to see that sex education is instituted on a broad basis. These goals are foremost in her words and work. They are grounded in the journey which brought Dr. Elders to the climax of her career. Her concerns and goals are undergirded in the values which Dr. Elders learned early on in life. Her work is about helping people to understand how to do and be, not what to do or be. She bases her work in a strong sense of values, rather than cheap, easy moralisms. She believes strongly that we should have a keen sense of values which provide us the foundation for making choices for our lives. Her opponents espouse a set of moralisms which allow no room for choices, but which offer clear cut, rigid rules for how to behave in any given situation. Dr. Elders understands that life is simply not that clear cut. Her understanding of the complexity of life includes the belief that we must look realistically at our situations and take responsibility for addressing current problems and working for a better future. The programs she advocates, her words and work exemplify this belief. This is what makes her controversial. It is also what helped her to withstand the claims and charges of her opponents during the confirmation process.

The Waiting is Over—Or Is It?

The hearing before the Senate Committee on Labor and Human Resources had been re-scheduled to commence on Friday morning, July 23, 1993. I got up early that morning after a restless night spent thinking about what more could happen to my sister during the Confirmation process. The family members who had returned to Washington to give support during the hearings all stayed in a number of rooms Dr. Elders had reserved for us in the Washington Holiday Inn Downtown. Dr. Elders had called and made all the arrangements for those family members who wanted to come and be there for the hearing.

Our family will always be indebted to the management and staff of the Washington Holiday Inn Downtown for the kind hospitality and assistance they provided Dr. Elders during the three months she stayed there while working at the Department of Health and Human Resources while waiting to go through the Confirmation process for the post of Surgeon General. The management and staff went all out to make sure the hotel lived up to the motto of being the "Nation's number one, or best, innkeeper." All the hotel employees seemed to have taken a personal role in making sure Dr. Elders was safe and comfortable. During the Confirmation process, the staff, and even some of the guests at the Hotel, would tell her to "hang in there, Dr. Elders." As the African proverb says, "It takes the whole village to raise a child." The people at the Holiday Inn Downtown became that village for Dr. Elders and her family during the Confirmation process. And I can truly say after going through the Confirmation process with my sister, it takes a whole nation of loving, caring and wonderful people to get a controversial "lightning rod" like Dr. Elders confirmed.

After I completed my walk around the Washington Mall that Friday morning (the Mall was two blocks over from the Hotel) I stopped by a Roy Rogers Restaurant to pick up breakfast for Joycelyn, Oliver and myself. Dr. Elders was up early making preparations for her testimony before the Senate Committee. As I sat there that morning I thought about a thousand things I wanted to say to help her get through the day, but I could only bless the food and whisper a breath prayer, "Lord, help us to hold out."

The Presidential Assistant who directs public liaison and staff, Alexis Herman, called and told Dr. Elders that our transportation to the Senate hearing would pick us up about 8:30 a.m. We finished our preparations and were ready to go when they picked us up. When we arrived at the building for the hearing, a number of Dr. Elders' supporters were outside the building holding up signs and cheering her on. I thought to myself, that maybe the Lord had called her to the Washington political kingdom for such a time as this. When we arrived in the room where the hearing was to take place, we found many friends from Arkansas and across the country who had come to Washington to support my sister. As we approached the hour when the Confirmation hearing was to begin, we found out that the Republicans, following the leadership of Don Nickles of Oklahoma, had pulled another stall tactic and delayed the hearing process yet again. Don Nickles had invoked a rule of the Senate which said that hearings could not take place while the Senate was in session. The rule was meant to insure that all Senators would be present in the Senate during crucial voting times; that morning was not an especially crucial voting time in the Senate. Senator Kennedy commented on the delay during the brief thirty minute session of the Committee that morning before the Senate went into session,

> *When you have an individual as distinguished as Dr. Elders, who has been honored by the President of the United States by nominating her to a position of enormous importance to the American people, when public health issues cry out for attention and leadership, to have a parliamentary procedure used to deny the full opportunity for this committee to hold its examination of the wide range of public policy issues involved and of the charges which have been leveled against Dr. Elders — and when Dr. Elders is denied the opportunity to present her case to the public — I think it is a shame for this institution to have that kind of policy. But it does exist, and quite frankly, we are going to deal with it in the only way that we know how, and that is with fairness to the nominee.*
>
> *So I would suggest to all of my colleagues on this committee that they cancel whatever plans they might have had through the afternoon, through the evening and through tomorrow, because that is the way that we are going to proceed on this committee. I am not going to be part of an effort to put this over for another day or for another week, to permit scurrilous accusations to be made against this nominee without an opportunity to respond. (U.S. Gov't Printing Office, S.Hrg.103-628, 2)*

Senator Kennedy moved the short morning session along in order to allow as much to be done as possible between 9:35 when they convened and 10:10 a.m. when they were forced to recess. During this short morning session there were accusations passed back and forth between Senator Coats and others on the Committee during which Senator Coats made the statement that *"there ought to be a full and fair and objective, thorough discussion of issues that have been raised mostly by the media and not members of the Republican party..."* (U.S. Gov't Printing Office, S.Hrg. 103-628, 2). It seemed to me that the media had not dreamed up these charges and that the media certainly hadn't been the ones to delay the hearing process. Again I marveled at a call for objectivity from Senator Coats, one of the least objective people on the committee, it seemed to me.

After the political wrangling was over, the hearing got on track with Dr. Elders' opening statement. Dr. Elders was interrupted once during her statement when the hour came for the hearing to recess because the Senate was going into session. Senator Kennedy held the hearing over for the additional time needed for Dr. Elders to complete her statement. Dr. Elders was invited to first introduce her family and then to give her statement.

"Many say I am a lightening rod. Please know that they [family and friends] have been my thunder" (U.S. Gov't Printing Office, S.Hrg. 103-628, 10). Dr. Elders prefaced her opening statement to the Committee with these words. They show her understanding of herself as one who takes the risk to say the things that need to be said which often draw a lot of heat, and it shows that she understands that it is her background and the support of her family and friends that allows her to do this. She went on in her statement to highlight the themes that she considers crucial to improve the state of health care in our country. Her general themes were: the need for health education and preventive health care; the need to look for and make the most of opportunities that we have and seeing that our children are provided with opportunities; her role as provider, teacher, scientist, administrator and coalition builder. She developed these

themes in the body of her statement and addressed many of the issues raised by her opponents. I believe her words speak best for her. The body of her opening statement follows below.

> *I appear before you today at a time when our entire nation is facing great challenges in public health. AIDS, violence, teenage pregnancy, a drug resistant strain of tuberculosis, low immunization rates all indicate we have not done a very good job at selling healthy lifestyles in this country. I believe the only way to heal our nation is through prevention. Prevention requires education. If confirmed, I would make my utmost goal the education of our people, all our people, on how to stay healthy.*
>
> *I have some personal and professional understanding of these challenges that I would like to share with you.*
>
> *I am the oldest of eight children. I had never seen a physician prior to my first year at college. One of my earliest memories concerning the lack of health care was my 4-year old brother, who had a ruptured appendix and was taken to the doctor more than ten miles away on the back of a mule. His abdomen was lanced, a drain placed, and he was sent home. I have heard my mother scream during difficult child deliveries without any medical help. I have seen bright young people all over this country surrounded by social problems impacting health such as drugs, alcohol, violence, homicide, suicide, AIDS and teen-age pregnancy. My experience has led me to know first-hand many of the programs administered by the Public Health Service and other federal agencies.*
>
> *Second, I know about taking advantage of opportunities. The United Methodist Church helped me to reach the first rung of the ladder that enabled me to be here today by providing a scholarship to Philander Smith*

College at age 15. After college, I enlisted in the Army and became a physical therapist. Following my service years, I attended medical school on the GI Bill and after completing my medical training became a board certified pediatric endocrinologist. I know the importance of providing opportunities for our children today.

Third, as a physician in public health clinics and at the University of Arkansas School of Medicine, I have been the provider of many of the services supported by public health programs.

Fourth, I am a teacher. For over twenty years, I have been on the faculty in the department of pediatrics at the University of Arkansas School of Medicine.

During my medical career, I was a National Institutes of Health career development awardee. I served on NIH study sections, advisory committees for both the NIH and the FDA, and, as a consultant to or as a member of advisory committees for many of the programs sponsored by the Public Health Service. I am an experienced researcher, having authored many articles on hormonal growth disorders in children. I appreciate the need to have good scientific facts to back up conclusions.

For the past five and a half years, I have been an administrator at the state level as Director of the Arkansas Department of Health. Last year, I was honored by my fellow Health Directors when they elected me President of the Association of State and Territorial Health Officers (ASTHO).

Finally, I am a coalition builder. Since becoming the director of the Arkansas Department of Health, I have spent a great deal of my time recruiting the help of churches, schools, civic organizations, judges, businesses and local communities. I realized that I could not do the job alone. I needed to mobilize all of the resources available in our communities to help save the most valuable resources we will ever have, our human capital. I do not believe that we can dictate from above what local communities need to do to solve the public health problems we are encountering today. We must empower each community to design their own solutions.

As a result of my background, education, training, and experience, I have become a strong advocate for programs that will strengthen families, reduce risky behaviors, improve health and enable children to become healthy, educated, motivated and to have hope for the future. Far too many of our children have become members of what I call the 5-H Club: hungry, healthless, homeless, hugless, and hopeless.

I would like to explain what I am about. But before I do that I would like to address some issues about me that have been raised.

I am about early childhood education to help children get a good start in life. Only 18 percent of Medicaid children in Arkansas, the poorest of the poor, have the opportunity to attend Headstart. We know that early childhood education is cost-effective and a preventive measure that reduces the likelihood that such children will end up as dropouts, in prison, or as teen parents.

I am about, and always have been about, comprehensive health education from kindergarten through the 12th grade. Comprehensive health education means age-appropriate health education programs which include information on nutrition, exercise, violence prevention, AIDS and human sexuality. It means being healthy and feeling good about yourself. Comprehensive health edu-

cation teaches children to take care of themselves. Our children deserve that choice.

I advocate educating our parents so that all will know how to instill in their children the courage, strength and perseverance to meet the challenges of growing up. We do not teach parents how to be good parents. Because they do not want to do anything wrong, too often some parents simply do nothing when it comes to providing sound, solid direction and guidance for their children.

I believe we must teach our young men to be responsible. Children being born today need all the help they can get to succeed in this world: including two nurturing parents when possible. They deserve to know and receive support from both parents. Young men must learn that being a father is more than just donating sperm.

I am about comprehensive school-based or school-linked health services which provide primary preventive care for children at or near where they spend most of their day, in school. In Arkansas, it was my policy (which was later codified) that the local community and the local elected school board would decide if they wanted a clinic in their school and what services to be provided in the clinic. Only four out of 24 clinics in Arkansas offer contraceptives on site. Even in those clinics, the parents must sign a release statement before their child can receive family planning counseling and contraceptives from the clinic.

I believe we must offer our bright, young people hope for the future by providing scholarships to those who stay out of trouble and do well in school so they can attend college. It is far cheaper to send them to college than to send them to prison.

Finally, I am about improving the quality of life of all

Americans by:

Preventing chronic and infectious diseases, including cancer, heart disease, hypertension, tuberculosis and AIDS.
Reducing infant morbidity and mortality.
Eliminating the serious disparities in health problems that minority groups experience.
Preventing and reducing the toll of injuries and disabilities in our society.
Improving women's health.
And providing care and services for our elderly so they can live in dignity and comfort during their final years.

As surgeon general, I will be a true advocate for the improvement of health in America, a strong, dedicated leader for the U.S. Public Health Service Commissioned Corps and an effective representative for the Public Health Service.

Mr. Chairman and members of the committee, I want to change the way we think about health by putting prevention first. I want to change the behaviors and attitudes of Americans by promoting programs and policies which will enable us to be responsible for our own health. I want to be the voice and the vision for the poor and powerless. I want to change concern about social problems that affect health into commitment. And I would like to make every child born in America a planned, wanted child.

Should I be confirmed, I would like to work with you and all America to develop an action plan to improve the health of our country. To me, it is not enough to just reform the health-care system. We will never have a large enough budget to address all the health-care needs of our citizens if we do not start thinking prevention and taking personal responsibility for our health.

I am a hard worker. I am willing to give my time and talent. We have a big task before us, and I hope you will see fit to make me part of your team.... (U.S. Gov't Printing Office, S.Hrg. 103-628, 10-12)

In this statement Dr. Elders makes it perfectly clear what she stands for and why. The things she stands for are issues which need immediate and radical attention if our children are to have any kind of future at all. To say that her stands are too controversial is to say that we refuse to address the crises we face in our country today. To say that her programs, words and work are too radical is to say that we would rather remain passive and let the future take care of itself, which it is doing as our society slowly self-destructs before our eyes because of the AIDS epidemic and the spread of other infectious diseases, rising teenage pregnancy, drug and other substance abuse, the increase of violence, poverty and the lack of preventive health care and education. Dr. Elders' words to the Senate Committee show her concerns and commitment to try to do something about making a better future for our children and our country. Her opponents, however, remained vigilant in their attempt to keep her from moving ahead.

One of the high points of the hearings came during Joycelyn's opening statement when she broke down and started to cry after she told about my father taking our four year old brother Bernard ten miles on the back of a mule to a doctor for a ruptured appendix. I was afraid, because I had never seen my oldest sister cry before. However, she quickly regained her composure and proceeded on with her statement. I remembered that Carl T. Rowan had written in his book *"Breaking Barriers"* that President Lyndon Johnson had told him, *"Carl, a man ain't worth a good god-*

damn if he can't cry at the right time" (261). Or, as the writer of Ecclesiastes wrote, *"To everything there is a season, and a time to every purpose under the heaven... A time to weep, and a time to laugh; a time to mourn and a time to dance"* (Ecclesiastes 3:1, 4 KJV).

Dr. Elders completed her opening statement at 10:10 a.m. and Senator Kennedy was forced to recess the hearing until after the Senate completed its business for the day. This meant another waiting period before the committee could begin its work in earnest. During this delay, we were invited to wait in the office of Senator Edward Kennedy. Our family will never be able to repay Senator Kennedy for the hard work and many, many hours he spent in making preparations to lead Dr. Elders through the Confirmation process. I had not met Senator Kennedy in person before that day, but when I met him, I was very impressed and felt that he truly is a giant of a man.

Finally at 1:05 that afternoon the stalling tactics of the Republicans had run out and the Confirmation hearing was re-called to order by Senator Kennedy. After a number of Senators from both parties, and Representative Blanche Lambert from Arkansas, had spoken in support of her, Dr. Elders responded to questions put to her. She would testify for four hours before the Committee. During those hours before the Senate Labor and Human Resources Committee, Dr. Elders refused to recant or back away from what she had said and done while she was the Director of Health for the State of Arkansas.

As expected Dr. Elders was asked questions about her bank dealings, the social security taxes for her mother-in-law's nurse, the recall of a batch of condoms from Arkansas clinics, her role in the Public Health Services and about all the quotations that had been pulled out of context and used against her by her opponents. She remained constant in her answers, again and again explaining that she is about preventive health care and education, but that she refuses to ignore the difficult issues which confront our country because they make some uncomfortable by naming them. The overwhelming majority of the committee members were strong in their support of Dr. Elders and in stating over and over that they believed that she was what our country needed: a Surgeon General who was not afraid to address head-on the hard issues, without regard to political correctness. I think that Senator Metzenbaum's words during his allotted time give a good flavor of the support Dr. Elders' received from the majority of the committee. Rather than asking questions, Senator Metzenbaum summarized his feelings about the process. He said that he was concerned over the seemingly inordinate amount of time spent on the issues of the bank and the social security, *"there has been more to-do about this...than maybe has been warranted"* (U.S. Gov't Printing Office, S.Hrg. 103-628, 43). Senator Metzenbaum stated his belief in Dr. Elders' integrity and went on to say to Dr. Elders, *"You are an unbelievably capable, aggressive, aggressive woman, and I think that's what we need in fighting some of the problems in this country"* (44). This support for Dr. Elders was unequivocal and not contingent upon her being politically correct. On the contrary, Senator Metzenbaum's support was based on the very fact that he believed Dr. Elders would be *"a breath of fresh air... [who was] going to do a fantastic job for the health care needs of this country"* (44).

The tense moments during the hearing came, as expected, during the questioning by Senator Coats. He spent a majority of his allotted time on the financial aspects of Dr. Elders' record and on a select few comments pulled out of context. At several points during his questioning he was interrupted by Senator Kennedy in order to allow Dr. Elders to clarify her comments and to keep Coats from misinterpreting her words. During one of Senators Coats' questioning periods he and Dr. Elders had a rather comical exchange. Senator Coats began by thanking Senator Durenberger for some "nice things" spoken about him during Senator Durenberger's turn. Dr. Elders responded, *"Senator, I thought you were very nice when I came to visit you, so I have been saying nice things about you, too"* (U.S. Gov't Printing Office, S.Hrg.103-628, 69). This exchange epitomizes Joycelyn Elders. Even though Senator Coats had been a major opponent, in my estimation an enemy, Joycelyn was able to say something good about, and to, him. This graciousness is sometimes overlooked, or overwhelmed, by the picture of the aggressive woman who fights for the health of our nation.

The hearing moved rather smoothly in the afternoon session, once all the delay-tactics were exhausted. By 4:54 that afternoon the questions and answers were complete, except for the written questions which would be submitted to Dr. Elders for a written response. Senator Kennedy concluded by saying that he thought the hearing had been *"an extraordinary exposition on public health"* and that he looked forward to having a *"Surgeon General who has the breadth of experience and the deep, deep commitment"* of Dr. Elders (U.S. Gov't Printing Office, S.Hrg. 103-628, 83).

The Battle is Won, but the War is Not Over

Following the hearing, Dr. Elders' nomination to be America's top doctor proceeded to the Senate floor for debate and final confirmation. Again there was a delay in bringing the nomination to the Senate floor, but debate finally began there on September 7, 1993. After the nomination was officially read for the record, Senator Kennedy proceeded to speak first on Dr. Elders' behalf. In his statement urging that Dr. Elders be confirmed as "the family doctor to the Nation," Senator Kennedy describes Dr. Elders in the following way,

> Dr. Elders is not anti-Catholic. She is not a radical. She is not outside the mainstream. She is not a divisive person. She is a healer and coalition builder who has worked with a wide variety of people of diverse viewpoints to being better health care to the people of Arkansas and the Nation. Most of all, she is a preacher and a teacher of immense commitment and knowledge – exactly what we need in a Surgeon General, America's First Physician. (U.S. Cong. Joint Committee on Printing S10980, S10981)

Senator Kennedy correctly characterizes Dr. Elders and understands that she is immanently qualified to address the vital issues of health care in our country. The issues were defined by Senator Kennedy in his statement as being children who are denied a "healthy start in life," infant mortality, childhood vaccinations, drugs, crime, violence, teenage pregnancy, health care for senior citizens, lack of adequate preventive care, women's health, AIDS, tuberculosis and the fact that "*in all areas of health care it is the poor and minorities who suffer the most*" (U.S. Cong. Joint Committee on Printing S10980). These are exactly the issues Dr. Elders has sought to address and they are the issues her critics have been quick to bring up in their opposition against her. Kennedy says of her opponents that they,

> ...have left no stone unturned in their unseemly attempt to undermine her record and character. The allegations against her have proved groundless in every case. Her opponents have distorted her record and twisted her statements into an unrecognizable caricature of the nominee. We are voting today on the real Dr. Elders, not the straw woman her opponents have attempted to portray. (U.S. Cong. Joint Committee on Printing S10980-10981)

Senator Kennedy goes on to say that those who have

opposed Dr. Elders basically have attacked her on two fronts, abortion and teen pregnancy (U.S. Joint Committee on Printing S10981). He appreciates the fact that these two issues are vitally important to our country and that no effective Surgeon General can be soft on these issues. We cannot afford any longer to not take a clear, decisive and active stand to see that the rise of unwanted, unloved, and poorly cared for children is stopped. Senator Kennedy understands that Dr. Elders stands for something, not simply against what are perceived as "moral evils." It is this sort of strong and committed person who can make a difference, even in Washington, if given the opportunity and support. Senator Kennedy strongly favored Dr. Elders for this reason.

A number of other Senators, likewise, rose in support of Dr. Elders on the Senate floor. Some twenty-one Senators spoke in favor of Dr. Elders' confirmation and twelve spoke against. In the debate on the Senate floor the same issues were raised and countered as had been raised in the hearing before the Senate Committee. No one tried to refute the fact that Dr. Elders is a very outspoken advocate for the programs she believes are necessary to change the current tide of health care in America. In fact, it is her outspokenness which drew the opposition of her critics. It remains, however, as Senator Moseley-Braun said in her comments,

> ...that we are now going to judge nominees not only based on their credentials and their competence and their character, but we are now going to base them on whether or not their quotations fit with our view of what people should and should not say.... [Y]ou can only talk about issues in a way that sounds good, that does not ruffle feathers, that does not displease people, does not put people off because, if you do, you stand in grave danger of having someone stand on the floor of the Senate and ques-

tion your commitment because of the way that you make your statements. *(U.S. Joint Committee on Printing S10988)*

This is the reason Dr. Elders' fitness for the job of Surgeon General was questioned, simply because there were those who did not like the way she said what she said. At least, she was willing to say something, unlike most of the politicians in Washington who talk continually, but say nothing of any account and do even less. Senator Boxer recognized this fact as she spoke in support of Dr. Elders, saying,

> *...when we do speak out clearly on these very tough issues, just by the very nature of the subject we are discussing we are being controversial. And certainly in the area of public health — preventing teen pregnancy, preventing teen suicide, preventing AIDS and other sexually transmitted diseases — we must not be afraid to be tough and controversial. We finally have someone, it seems to me, who is not afraid to stand up and tell it like it is, as painful as it may be.*
>
> *Many times... the world is not the way we want it to be, or we would hope it would be, or we wish it would be. We must deal with it as it is presented to us, and sometimes these subjects are very difficult.*
>
> *...We have discussed her qualifications at length and the support that she has at length. But I want to concentrate in the remainder of my remarks on the three main reasons I find to support Dr. Elders. They are as follows: our children, our children, our children.*
>
> *We know that Dr. Elders has offended some members of this body, and they have been very eloquent in their critique of her. They are offended by some of her words.*

> But, again, I must point out that we need to be at least as offended by the status of our children. And... I say to you if we are as offended by the status of our children as by some of the things she said, we would have voted to confirm Dr. Elders long ago.
>
> ...So let us not waste any more time.... Let us get with it.... We are hearing the same things over and over and over again.... I defend every Senator's right to say anything he wants to or she wants to over and over, but to what end at this point? Let us vote. Let us change the status of our children. Let us give our children hope. Let us attack these problems in a direct way for the health of our children and our country. (U.S. Joint Committee on Printing S10998, 10999)

Senator Boxer heard Dr. Elders' call to action and issued one to the Senate. This is what it will take for the trend to change in our nation. Indeed, if our children are to have a future, this sort of call must be raised from the rooftops across our country.

The debate on the Senate floor, as well as the hearing before the Committee, were as Senator Boxer characterized them, "the same things over and over and over again." It seemed no one had any new issues to raise, that no one had any real ammunition in their attacks on Dr. Elders other than personal ideology. Senator Bumpers aptly described the entire process when he said in his remarks,

> Nobody is arguing with the truthfulness of what she has said. They are arguing with her indiscretion and lack of diplomacy in saying things that need to be said. Harry Truman, one of the five greatest Presidents of this country, did not know the meaning of diplomacy. But make no mistake about it, when he said it, everybody knew what he was talking about.... (U.S. Joint Committee on Print-

ing S11009)

> [Dr. Elders] *says things bluntly. I wish at times like this she were not quite so blunt. But I promise you that all these Senators who have been off on this August recess making speeches at various places, hear in townhall meetings: "Why don't you politicians tell it like it is? Why can't you say what you mean and mean what you say?" Or as Senator Herman Talmadge used to say, "You have to throw the corn where the hogs can get to it." You have to say it so the least among us can understand what you are saying. (U.S. Joint Committee on Printing S11008)*

Indeed, this is what Dr. Elders has done, said things so they could be understood. However, it seems that often what has happened is what Jesus referred to as "casting your pearls before swine" (Matthew 7:6). Often those listening have been stopped by the way Dr. Elders says the difficult things she does and they have failed to hear what she was saying and to recognize its vital importance. Another of the sayings of Jesus comes to mind, -"those who have ears to hear, let them hear" (Matthew 13:9 NRSV).

The Summit in View

When Dr. Elders' confirmation finally came to a vote, the result was 65 to 34 in favor of confirmation, with the votes divided largely along party lines. I had sat and watched through the hearing and through the debate on the floor. I had heard my sister's words and work run through the wringer, and I felt that the confirmation had been too long in coming. I looked forward to what lay ahead for Dr. Elders and I believed that she would make positive advances in the state of public health in our country. I also knew that the road which lay ahead would not be any easier than the one down which she had come. I hoped that Senator Kennedy's words from his opening statement would prove to be true, "*Now, the Nation as a whole is about to feel the healing touch of this extraordinary woman. In the years to come it may well be said of Joycelyn Elders, as it was of Franklin Roosevelt, that she is loved for the enemies she made*" (U.S. Cong. Joint Committee on Printing S10981).

Chapter Fifteen

SHORT-LIVED SUMMIT—NO PLACE TO REST

> *But you rise up against my people as an enemy;*
> *you strip the robe from the peaceful,*
> *from those who pass by trustingly with no thought of war.*
> *The women of my people you drive out from their pleasant houses;*
> *from their young children you take away my glory forever.*
> *Arise and go;*
> *for this is no place to rest,*
> *because of uncleanness that destroys with a grievous destruction.*
> *If someone were to go about uttering empty falsehoods, saying,*
> *'I will preach to you of wine and strong drink,'*
> *such a one would be the preacher for this people!*
> Micah 2:8-11 NRSV

Surgeon General Elders

Dr. Elders' reached what seemed the summit of her career by winning confirmation as the first Black and second woman Surgeon General. It seemed that she had finally arrived at the pinnacle and could enjoy going about her work and making a difference in public health for the whole country. The task before her was no small one, but she, being no stranger to hard work, set out determinedly to do the very best job she could to make the most difference in the lives of as many people as possible. Being a good United Methodist, Dr. Elders lives by John Wesley's admonition to, "do all the good you can, to all the people you can, in all the places you can, for just as long as you can" (Outler 249). She was determined to do just that.

The office of Surgeon General has had a varied history. It began in 1871 and had a period of years when no one held the office. The Surgeon General in recent history has been responsible for managing the Public Health Service's Commissioned Corps. The Surgeon General receives the military rank of three-star admiral. In her position as Surgeon General, Dr. Elders' areas of responsibility included: PHS' Offices of Population Affairs, Minority Health, Women's Health, and the President's Council on Physical Fitness and Sports. The real responsibility Dr. Elders would have as Surgeon General was to make a difference in the health of a whole nation. This was no small task and one which, because of the nature of the office of Surgeon General, would not be quickly or easily accomplished. The Surgeon General of the United States, while the office has been around over a century, has little real power — at least not as power is measured in Washington. John Schwartz characterized the office quite aptly in an July 16, 1993 article in *The Washington Post*, the same article Dr. Elders had shown us when Coach Elders and I arrived for the first hearing date. Schwartz wrote,

> *The top uniformed official of the Public Health Service does not have a lot of institutional power. The surgeon general is, essentially, the federal official who tells people to eat their peas and to live right. Surgeons general, for example, might wish to wage war on cigarettes — Koop and his successor Antonia C. Novello certainly did — but the only weapon they have is their mouths. (A7.1)*

Of course, Dr. Elders was perhaps better armed in this wise than some others; perhaps, in retrospect, it seems she was too well-armed. She was prepared and committed to speak out on the issues that she knows from experience are crucial for our country. She understood her job as Surgeon General was, as she said in an interview two days after her confirmation in the Senate, *"to articulate, promote and lobby for sound health policy"* (Hilts C9.2)

At her swearing in on September 8, 1993 Dr. Elders became the sixteenth person to hold the office of Surgeon General. As Surgeon General she was entrusted with the task of carrying out the mission of the Public Health Service, *"improving and advancing the health of our Nation's people"* (U.S. Dept. of Health and Human Services 1). She approached this job committed to do her best. A little ragged from the confirmation process, her devotion to the task of improving our nation's health was not daunted. She spoke with President Clinton shortly after the approving vote by the Senate. During the conversation President Clinton expressed his pleasure about the victory and even about the hard-fought confirmation battle. Dr. Elders replied to him, in her typical style, *"Well, I'm glad you enjoyed it. Things have not really gone too smoothly. I came to Washington as prime steak, and after being there a little while I feel like low-grade hamburger"* (Hilts C1.1). However, she still set out with her usual determined spirit to do the best job she knew how.

Dr. Elders had clearly spelled out during her confirmation process what her priorities would be as Surgeon General. As always, she was about preventive health care, health education and making a better future for our children. As she said in her testimony during the Confirmation hearing,

> *"I want to change the way we think about health by putting prevention first. I want to change the behaviors and attitudes of Americans by promoting programs and policies which will enable each of us to be responsible for our own health. I want to be the voice and the vision of the poor and the powerless. I want to change concern about social problems that affect health into commitment. And I would like to make every child born in America a*

planned and wanted child. (U.S. Gov't Printing Office, S.Hrg. 103-628, 12)

This is no small task she set for herself, but it is one that she set right to work on. Certainly the changing of attitudes, behavior and "concern" to "commitment" is a long and arduous process. It is perhaps easier to simply implement new programs than to change people's minds. As the old saying goes, "it is always easier to ask forgiveness than permission." However, what Dr. Elders understands is that any real change in the state of public health in our country will take more than simply implementing a few new programs and spending a few billion more tax dollars. In order to make any real difference in our own lives now, or especially in our children's future, we must change the ways we think, which will directly change the ways we act. This is what Dr. Elders' seeks to do with her gospel of health care and education that she preached from the pulpit of the Surgeon General's office and which she is still going around the country preaching.

Part-time Prophet

Dr. Elders is a prophetic voice—but she is not simply a portent of doom. She offers ideas and programs which will make a difference. The things of which she speaks are not popular, and often not pleasant. But she has the guts and determination it takes to be a prophet who stands firm in her message and who offers us the tools to change. It is a curious tragedy that we will not listen to her, that our country refuses to hear this important message. Are we afraid? Are we too proud? Are we so naive as to believe that if we don't talk about it, it isn't real? Our society seems to be much like the family system of an addicted person. We all know the problem is there; we can all clearly see the damage being done. And yet, we all sit by in silence refusing to believe that this painful reality can actually be true in our family. These things happen to others, not to us. Maybe if we don't talk about it, it will go away. I think this is especially true for the attitudes of the "religious right." They seem especially unwilling to confront painful reality. They are the prophets of doom and the proponents of "pie-in-the-sky-by-and-by." They preach against everything and for very little except what a clergywoman colleague of mine called their shallow "Jesus-wejus'" (from "Jesus we jus' want... prayers) religion. Their "Jesus-wejus'" resembles very little the Christ of the Christian faith. He is against everything, according to them. From my reading of the Bible the only thing Jesus the Christ condemned was a pompous faith — like the Pharisees. But the mentality of the "religious right" is that we don't need to talk about the horrific realities of our society, we just need to talk about Jesus and "turn it all over to Jesus." It seems to me that Jesus the Christ called and commissioned disciples to go into a hurting world and continue his work of touching it where it hurts. That means being realistic about the problems that are there and addressing them in tangible ways. That is what Dr. Elders' work is all about. That is what her message is all about.

In a foreword to the Sonoma County Physician Dr. Elders says

> *Having been the Surgeon General for nearly a year now, I have come to realize that the job often requires me to speak about social and behavioral problems that impact health, problems which we as a nation prefer not to discuss. It meant talking to the American people about changing their behavior to prevent health problems before they occur. It means providing age appropriate comprehensive health education in our schools from kindergarten through 12th grade. We must teach our citizens how to be healthy and address the issue of responsible sexuality. The most common cause of death for*

> young men between the ages of 25-44 is AIDS. The largest risk-factor for poverty among children under six is to be born to an unmarried adolescent mother who has not finished high school.
>
> My primary goal as Surgeon General is the education of our people, all our people, on how to stay healthy. I want to change the way we think about health — by putting prevention first.
>
> To me, it is not enough just to reform the health care system or "sick care system;" we must also reform the public health and the community health systems. We will never have a large enough budget to address all the health care needs of our citizens if we do not start thinking about prevention and begin taking personal responsibility for our own health.... ("Sonoma County" 1)

Dr. Elders again and again has taken the message to anyone who would listen. Her concern is genuine for the people of this country. Her concern is greatest for the children of this country. President Clinton knew this when he nominated her to be Surgeon General. He knew this from working with her in Arkansas. One thing he learned about Dr. Elders while they worked together in Arkansas is that she is a tireless, outspoken worker who says and does what she feels is in the best interest of public health. He learned it the hard way on her first day as Director of the Arkansas Department of Health. On the day then-Governor Clinton announced her appointment to the state position, Dr. Elders was asked by a reporter about whether she planned to distribute condoms. She replied with the now famous quote, *"Well, we won't be putting them on their lunch trays, but yes."* As David Nimmons writes about this incident in *Playboy*, *"The governor cringed, turned red, gulped several times — then gamely stood by his choice. The public Dr. Elders — corrupter of youth, scourge of the right — was born"* (56). Dr. Elders was upfront from the very first day in public, political life and she remains so today. She continually proved this in the short time she held the office of Surgeon General. Unfortunately there are too many who are not ready or willing to hear the truth that Dr. Elders speaks. What she says is not "politically correct" in the sense that she doesn't worry about whose political toes are stepped on when it comes to what is best for this country and public health. She is very much like the ancient Hebrew prophets who spoke messages that were none too welcome by those at whom they were directed. As in the quotation from Micah at the beginning of this chapter, Dr. Elders knows that there are many who rise up against the people of God as an enemy, especially against the poor, children, minorities, unwed mothers, persons with AIDS, homosexuals and the list goes on. Like in Micah's day, there are those who seek to "strip the robe" from those who stand up for the rights of the needy. Women and children today, as is Micah's time, are still often the victims. People would still rather hear a messenger who preaches the wantonness of the status-quo rather than the radical gospel of change. Dr. Elders knows that "this is no place to rest." She understands that there is no rest until there is change for the better. Dr. Elders knows no other message than that radical message of change — the only message which holds any hope for our nation. She was tireless in her tenure as Surgeon General, and she is still not resting, but is tirelessly continuing to preach her radical gospel. She prophesies the doom which awaits us if we do not change the course of health care in our country and she offers us ways to do so.

Perhaps Dr. Elders' statement published in *USA Today* on December 12, 1994 best summarizes her short-lived summit and explains why there is for her still "no place to rest."

I have been honored to serve this country and this President as Surgeon General of the United States Public Health Service. I have followed the tradition of this office by speaking out about the difficult choices we face in doing the right thing to keep our children and our country healthy.

My tenure, like that of many previous Surgeons General, has been marked by controversy. In accepting this job, I was well aware that conflict goes with the territory. Thus, the 1964 and 1986 reports on smoking of the Surgeons General Luther Terry and C. Everett Koop generated bitter debates. As with smoking, many public health issues are tough and complicated and involve intensely personal matters.

I also have spoken out on a number of pressing public health issues of the decade, which have made many people uncomfortable. At a time when our streets and jails are full of children nobody wants, and the rate of sexually transmitted diseases is growing, our country must find ways to attack these scourges. This means telling the truth to our young people about the risks of their behavior and giving them the means to reduce these risks.

In a society where nearly half of all poor children do not grow up in a conventional family structure, local communities and governments often end up playing surrogate parental roles. This is not because government is supposed to play parent; it is because there are sadly often no parents there. We come into the world alone, and we leave it alone. But, if we are fortunate, as I have been, we have families who love us and carry us through our darker days.

When working at its best, public health is invisible. It keeps babies healthy, our water clear of contamination, our children free from lead poisoning, gunshots, child abuse, AIDS, smoking and faulty immunization, and helps make every child a wanted and planned child.

During my short tenure, this administration has made enormous strides. In Minnesota a waterborne epidemic that killed 100 people was ended after public health officials identified the culprit. Lead poisoning of children is now at the lowest point in U.S. history because lead has been virtually removed from the gasoline supply. Deaths due to homicides have begun to drop in many cities because federal controls on assault weapons have finally been adopted. The rate of pregnancy in very young teenagers has also begun to fall, along with smoking by African-Americans.

I will continue to be a voice for the poor and the powerless and do my best to see that the goals of this administration are reached to make the world a better place for all of God's children. Godspeed to the President, new Congress and my colleagues as they continue to grapple with these matters. I pray that we all learn to lower the volume and raise the tolerance and wisdom of our public discussions. If I have saved the life of a single child, or prevented the spread of AIDS to even one more person, it has all be worthwhile. (12A)

Dr. Elders' goal was to improve the plight of the people in our nation who are so desperately in need. There are many who refuse to believe these people are worthy of saving. The Congress is fighting hard to take away programs on which these people depend. This is not to say that Dr. Elders, or I, support the abuses of the welfare and public aide systems that go on. However, what Dr. Elders knows all too well is that the longer we refuse to acknowledge the very real problems which exist in our country, the worse those problems are going to become.

Simply by ignoring them, we cannot make them go away. By cutting welfare funding we cannot make poverty go away. By not talking about AIDS except to condemn those who have the disease we cannot find a cure. By simply arresting those we find selling or using drugs we do not make the problem of drug addiction go away. By passing laws to allow people to legally carry concealed weapons, or cutting funding for law enforcement we do not end violence. By cutting funding to education we do not do away with ignorance that breeds poverty. By condemning homosexuality and running them out of the military we cannot make all persons have a heterosexual orientation. In order to affect any real change we must begin to talk openly and honestly, we must be willing to invest the best of ourselves and our resources to reaching out a tangible helping hand to those who are truly in need. In order to change things in our country we must change the ways we think. We must take our blinders off and look realistically at our problems. We cannot improve our country by overlooking, or pushing out of sight, the poor, the powerless or the controversial. We can only truly improve our country by starting with those who have the greatest needs and then working our way up. Dr. Elders understands this and this is what she worked so hard as Surgeon General to make people realize and what she continues to work for today.

Consciousness-Raiser

Even though she was Surgeon General for only some sixteen months, Dr. Elders did something to try and raise the consciousness of the country. She brought to our attention the crucial issues and crises which confront us today. Many may not have liked what they heard, but at least they heard. Perhaps, like the ancient Hebrews who listened to the prophets, if we hear long enough, the message will finally start to sink in. This is my hope and prayer, and Dr. Elders' hope, prayer and her relentless task. There is no place for any of us to rest as long as there are those among us who are in need. There is no place for any of us to rest as long as our country would rather condemn someone like Dr. Elders who is working to improve our country's health than condemn the causes of our societal crises. There is no real place to rest, even though there are many resting behind their stained-glass windows, closed office doors, closed drapes and blinds, closed minds. Dr. Elders is not resting, and will not rest until our country changes and the enemies — ignorance, poverty, sickness, violence, addiction, etc. — are defeated. The summit was short-lived and Dr. Elders continues to climb.

Chapter Sixteen

THE POLITICS OF DRUGS, RACE AND SEX

<u>"The Answer to a Riddle"</u>

One of the most celebrated riddles in all the world is that of the king who promised vast holdings to anyone who could answer this riddle: "What is it that does not change?"

It is said that after moments of silence, one of the king's wise men proclaimed that he had the answer, and proceeded to answer the king's riddle by saying, "Oh, King, change alone does not change." You see, hidden within the question lies part of the answer to the riddle. If the scene is changed from the king's court to America, what, then, is the answer to the riddle of politics, drugs, race and sex in America? Keep in mind that a riddle requires the correct answer, which is sometimes tricky.

On December 7, 1993 after delivering a speech to the National Press Club, a reporter asked Dr. Elders what she thought about the legalization of drugs in this country. In her reply she said, *"legalizing drugs* [she thought] *could markedly reduce the crime rate...."* However, Dr. Elders went on to say, *"but I don't know all of the ramifications of this and we need to do further studies...."*

After the renowned comment, Dr. Elders immediately came under fire from conservative and right-wing groups, including certain Republicans in the U.S. House of Representatives. Some of these individuals immediately called for her to resign as Surgeon General. As if that were not enough, it seems her immediate family also came under attack. Almost immediately following her comment to the National Press Club, her husband Oliver was attacked in the press concerning a rental house that the family owns in central Little Rock.

The Arkansas Democrat-Gazette reported in its December 11, 1993 issue that Elders' husband Oliver owned a rental house that neighbors contended was a hangout for gang members (Stumpe 1A, 16A). The Little Rock Police Department made an investigation of the neighbors' complaint and found no evidence to support the charge. We do not know the real motive behind the riddle of the neighbors' charge. However, we do know that a neighbor had tried to get Oliver to sell him the house at a reduced rate upon learning that the Elderses would be moving to Washington, D.C. We also know that after the damage to the family's credibility had been attempted, the young mother who lived in the house threatened to bring action against the City of Little Rock for false and untrue charges having been made. Not another word has been heard since then.

The answer to this riddle may be that the whole thing was a setup with the explicit purpose of embarrassing and eventually destroying the reputation of the Elderses as prominent public figures.

If the falsehood about the rental property were not enough, somewhat reminiscent of the story of Job in the Bible, the very next week the Little Rock Police issued a warrant charging Dr. Elders' twenty-eight year old son Kevin with one count of delivery of a controlled substance. The December 21, 1993 issue of the *Arkansas Democrat-Gazette* states that *"the warrant was issued nearly five months after a July 29, 1993 incident in which Kevin allegedly sold one-eighth ounce of cocaine to an undercover Little Rock Police narcotics officer for the amount of $275 in Boyle Park"* (Pincus B1.5). The riddle: "If this is true, why wasn't he charged instantly?"

The warrant was served eight days after Dr. Elders' statement to the National Press Club. The lead paragraph of the December 11, 1993 story in the *Arkansas Democrat-Gazette* smirked, "*For U.S. Surgeon General Joycelyn Elders, whose talk about drugs and violence sparked controversy in Washington this week, the problems may hit closer to her own home than she realized...*" (Stumpe 1A).

A police officer who assisted in the investigation said the timing of the warrant reflected normal procedure. Lt. Charles Holladay, a Little Rock Police Department official, claimed that the officers making the arrest were not aware that Kevin Elders was the son of the Surgeon General when they set up the drug buy (Pincus B1.5). I thought, "if you believe that, I have some ocean front property for sale in Pine Bluff, Arkansas, and I will also throw in the George Washington Bridge for free...."

We Stand By Our Son!

All children have a special place in the hearts of their parents, but very often it seems nothing can touch a mother's heart like a son, or a father's heart like a daughter. In ancient times we have the biblical story of King David's grief when he received the news that Joab had murdered his son Absalom. Showing his grief, King David is recorded to have screamed, "*Oh my son Absalom, my son, my son Absalom! Would God I had died for thee. O Absalom, my son, my son...*" (II Samuel 18:33, KJV).

The grief of the Elderses at the time they learned of the warrant for Kevin's arrest reminded me of King David's grief for Absalom. I remember the weekend well. I was home working in my office late one Sunday evening when I received a phone call from a reporter with United Press International inquiring about my knowledge of a "Kevin Maurice Elders." I told him that I knew a "Kevin Elders," my nephew, but that I did not know a "Kevin Maurice Elders." The reporter went on to inquire if I thought this Kevin Elders was my nephew. I replied that I had never heard him called "Kevin Maurice Elders." The reporter told me that the Little Rock Police were looking for him and had issued a warrant for his arrest charging him with one count of delivering a controlled substance. The reporter wanted to know if I had his telephone number or knew where he could be reached. I told him that I did not have my nephew Kevin's telephone number, but that I could give him his brother Eric's telephone number. The conversation terminated with my giving the reporter Eric's telephone number.

I immediately called my sister in Washington, D.C. to find out if the person being sought by the police could be Kevin. She told me that someone from the press had called her office and that the charge seemed to be about something that had occurred over five months prior to the time, and that in talking with Kevin he could not remember such an event taking place. She assured me that whatever the situation was, she and Oliver had retained a long time family friend, P.A. "Les" Hollingsworth, as legal counsel for Kevin.

As she moved toward the end of the discussion, I told her that I could not believe Kevin could be in any way identified with such a thing and that I believed the impending arrest was probably politically motivated and related to the comment she had made concerning the need to study the issue of legalizing drugs. At that point I also shared with her the fact that I had received a notice from the Internal Revenue Service stating that I owed nearly ten thousand dollars in back taxes. The notice was received the same day the police had issued the warrant from my nephew's arrest. I went on to say that I simply could not write off all of these events as coincidental.

Keep in mind that during this time the conservative and right-wing groups had heightened their call for President Clinton to fire Dr. Elders.

While I had her ear, I took full advantage of the opportunity. I told her that I thought all of these events (Kevin's arrest, the notice about my taxes, the attack on Oliver over the rent house and the increased call for her firing) were all racism and sexism clothed in what is called "politics," but the bottom line was a shrewdly planned effort to have her removed from office and out of Washington, D.C. In some quarters it is thought that in our society there is a support system for racism and sexism that pulls together to destroy anything or anyone "the system" perceives as a threat. Joycelyn, by this time sensing my anger, stopped me and said she did not believe these attacks were racially motivated. The real truth is she did not want to hear a lot of negative talk. All she wanted to do at this time was to be near and support her son, Kevin. The tone of her voice told me that she was thinking, "this, too, shall pass...." Thus, I tried to ease her pain and, at the same time, get a hold on my own frustration.

"The Things We Do For Love"

When the bottom drops out from under those we love we are willing to do many things out of our love. Kevin Elders is blessed with loving parents who have always cared for him, and who have been especially present in the most crucial times of his life. Joycelyn and Oliver have two wonderful sons, both of whom have been well-behaved their entire lives. In fact, on many occasions, the two have openly shared with others concerning how blessed they feel to have two wonderful sons. But, as is true of being parents, there have also been difficult times for them as a family.

Kevin has always had a problem with addiction. When he was a little boy he had an addiction problem with food. It is a well known fact that Kevin has fought obesity most of his life. His weight has always been a problem for him in many ways. The end result has been lowered self-esteem for him. The problem manifested itself especially during his teen years. It would worsen when he got to college and his substance of choice would change from food to smoking, alcohol, and, finally, marijuana and other drugs.

When Kevin was in the fifth grade, his parents sent him to a camp for obese children located in Stockbridge, Massachusetts. By this time Kevin weighed over two hundred pounds. The camp was good for him. He was glad to have other kids to play with. The experience at the camp was different from things back home in North Little Rock, Arkansas where the children teased him about his weight. The more he was teased, the more he ate; the more he ate, the worse he felt about himself.

At the camp, Kevin and his peers had something in common; they were all overweight. There no one picked on him. He felt good about himself. The children in the camp were placed on a 1500 calorie diet. People came from throughout the country to participate in the camp each summer. The counselors spent a great deal of time with the children, helping them to build higher self-esteem.

Tools for building higher self-esteem were what Kevin needed. Although he had a loving family, he needed some extra help in building his self-esteem. It is important that parents realize how crucial their role is in their children's self-image. The one gift which can enhance the self-esteem of children is the quality time spent with parents, guardians and caring adults. It is during this time that children learn that they are important as individuals. Parents today need to be very mindful of this need and to structure quality time with their children no matter what. Children today are facing many complex issues and problems which require them to be prepared early to make hard choices. Unfortunately, we know that too many of our young people are not able to deal with the tough situations. It seems that the bond of trust between children and their parents is being lost. For example, when many youths today find themselves faced with a choice of telling a lie, or the truth, many would rather lie, hoping the truth will never be known so they will not have to face the consequences of their actions. This renders parents impotent to help them, as they do not really understand the total picture of what has happened. Very often, the parents and children learn to distrust each other as a result. It only takes a little extra effort to prevent this from happening, a little extra attention: realizing that problems exist and seeking the best means to rectify the problems and equip children with the tools they need in life. Joycelyn and Oliver saw Kevin's need early on and sent him to the camp hoping to provide him with some of those needed extra resources.

Kevin's parents have always trusted him. The family has always been very close. They lived in good nurturing neighborhoods and the boys were surrounded with positive role models. They formed relationships with their neighbors. I recall a conversation with Kevin concerning a neighbor who was very special to him when the family resided in the Glenview Community in North Little Rock. The lady's name was Mrs. Byrd. He recalled how he would go to her house and she would give him treats. He said, "Mrs. Byrd made the best egg custard in the world!" To him, she was like another grandmother. She always had time for Kevin. He remembers her today as a very special person in his life.

Kevin also tells the story of something that happened when he was four or five years old. One day, while his parents and older brother slept, he walked from their home to Mrs. Byrd's stark naked. He said Mrs. Byrd, with a surprised look on her face, asked him, "Kevin, do your parents know that you are out like this?" He replied, "No," and she invited him inside while she called his parents and told them where he was and asked them to bring him some clothes.

This was the first time, Kevin says, that he realized the important social role that clothing played in covering one's body. This is probably true, because it was not unusual at all for him and his brother, while growing up, to walk about the house in their underwear. As Kevin shared this story with me, I related to him how uncomfortable it made me feel when I would come to visit the family and there he and Eric would be walking around in their underwear. I grew up in a more puritanical environment. We covered the body in the presence of others. Therefore, when I went to visit my sister in Little Rock and had my very first encounter with the boys walking around like that, I told them to go put on some clothes. They informed me that they had on clothing. I retorted, "No, you do not have on clothing, you have on underwear, and underwear is not considered clothing." The debate went on for a while and, finally, Joycelyn directed them to go and put their pants on for Uncle Chess. For me, this was when I started to notice a generation gap between the puritanical ways of my upbringing and the ways of the children who came along in the days of Woodstock in the 1960's. Things were different for the children who grew up then than they were for Joycelyn and me in our growing up years, and they are different now than they were in the 1960's. With each generation there are new issues and problems and concerns. It is our challenge to find the best ways to cope with today's situations and bring the best knowledge and experience from the past with us to meet today's needs.

The Move to Lakewood

Kevin and the Elderses moved from the Glenview Community to the Lakewood Subdivision, located in the rolling hills of North Little Rock near McCain Shopping Mall. The area was inhabited exclusively by whites before the Elderses moved in. The family enjoyed a pleasant reception and remained residents there for over twenty years before they moved to their present home on Marcia Cove in Little Rock.

Kevin recalls that the Lakewood neighborhood was nice; nevertheless, the only children he had to play with were white, and there were fewer children at that. He said the Lakewood and Glenview communities were different in that "the families were very close" in Glenview. "It was truly a community of neighbors; there were many friends and children with whom to play." He said he also missed the big garden the family had in Glenview. There wasn't room for such a garden at the Lakewood house. Kevin stated that he began to feel somehow less than the other children in the Lakewood community. He rationalized his feeling as being based on race. This feeling of being less because of his race may have played a part in other negative images Kevin developed. He later revealed that some of his old friends from the Glenview neighborhood would tease him at the Glenview Elementary School about living in a white neighborhood. Others would tease him about his weight. All of this was very difficult for a sixth grader who was still at the stage when he wanted to be liked by everyone.

To further complicate matters for Kevin, he noticed that his older brother, Eric, who had until then readily played with him and served as his protector in the community, now seemed not to want him around while he was with his friends. While this is natural among siblings at a certain age, Kevin internalized this as a rejection of him as a person.

While Kevin and Eric have always been very close as siblings, they do have different personalities. Eric has always seemed to have a zest for life and high self-esteem which Kevin lacked. His interest was body building, unlike Kevin who battled a weight problem. Eric began body building when he was very young, and today, at age thirty-one, could pass for a black Charles Atlas. He is very much at ease in almost any situation. He knows that he is somebody. He loves to work out each day at a fitness center, fish, hunt and teach school. It seems that life has somehow come easier to Eric than to Kevin.

Eric lives according to a strict ritual. He gets up each morning at 5:30 and goes to the gym to work out for an hour. He goes home to shower, dress, eat breakfast and is off to arrive at school early to start the day with the students. His students' parents have often marveled at how well Eric is able to relate to his students. Besides teaching and working out, Eric loves his quiet time at home, or on Lake Pine Bluff fishing. He is full of enthusiasm for life and loves the life he has made for himself, and his life is a contrast to Kevin's in many ways.

It is puzzling how two boys could have grown up in the same household, been raised by the same parents and yet be so different. I must say that neither of the boys gave their parents any trouble as youngsters, during high school, or immediately after leaving the nest to be out on their own. It was at some time during the college years that the two boys began asserting their very different personalities.

For Kevin, perhaps it all began after finishing high school. Only weeks after graduating from high school in 1983, Kevin checked into the hospital to have his stomach stapled as a weight control measure. Following the operation he had to adhere to a very restricted diet. Kevin now thinks the operation was a mistake. After having lost a great deal of weight following the operation, he continued to mentally envision himself as the same 340 pound person he had been before the operation. It seems this may have been the real beginning of his troubled young life which progressed to his present problem with drugs and alcohol. Actually, his trouble began while he was attending college at the University of Arkansas at Fayetteville. He said that when he had been overweight, although he suffered teasing about it at times, he really felt good on the inside and knew that his parents loved him. But, strangely enough, he somehow lost sight of this fact and began to turn to once again search for some measure of self-esteem.

Kevin has said that he was never really involved in drug use while in high school, except for the occasional sip of wine with friends during major school functions. He recounts that it was during his first semester at the University that he drifted into drugs and alcohol. During his first semester he shared an apartment with Eric. Eric had strict house rules which Kevin was expected to follow. Kevin said this made him feel like a child again, so he rebelled. He thinks it was a mistake to try and share an apartment with his brother. He soon moved out and into his own place for the second semester.

Kevin remained at the University for two and one-half years. Due to poor-self discipline and failing grades, Kevin dropped out of the University and returned to Little Rock. There he enrolled at his mother's alma mater, Philander Smith College. He did complete all requirements for his degree and graduated in the fall of 1988. Next Kevin enrolled at Grambling University as a graduate student. He received a Master's Degree in business administration in the Spring of 1990.

During the summer of 1990, Kevin returned to Little Rock and began to search for employment. This feat proved to be difficult, even with an MBA. While continuing his job search, he worked for his parents managing the family's rental properties. After waiting almost two years for even a good lead on a job, Kevin was hired by Johnson and Johnson Personal Products of North Little Rock in December, 1992. He worked there until his trial in 1994. Kevin had a good work record with the company and received praise from co-workers for his work as a night shift supervisor.

One-Half Teaspoon of Joy — An Ocean of Trouble

On July 1, 1993, President Clinton had officially nominated Kevin's mother to be U.S. Surgeon General. At almost the same time, a paid informant of the Little Rock Police Department, named Calvin Walraven, identified Herbert Jones, Jr. and Kevin as drug suppliers. Kevin had met Calvin Walraven at a Christmas party in 1990. The two became friends and, during the next two years, frequently met and shared pot and cocaine.

Calvin Walraven had a history of mental problems, drug abuse and, like Kevin, he had a weight control problem. When Calvin Walraven submitted to becoming a police informant, he was down on his luck and allegedly HIV positive. His friends had moved away from him. He was without work or a place to live. Walraven had become a person who had made a complete wreck of his life. In a way he had become like the biblical character, Esau, who was willing to sell his birthright and betray his friends for a mess of, in Calvin's case, "pot"tage.

On July 18, 1994, Walraven testified in Judge Plegge's court that he called Kevin every day during the month of July, 1993. This was immediately after Joycelyn had been nominated as Surgeon General. Finally, on July 28, 1993, Kevin agreed that he would get Walraven some "coke." Allegedly, the next day, Kevin met Walraven in Boyle Park while Little Rock Police detectives looked on. The transaction was allegedly made with money the police had given Walraven. Kevin was totally unaware that his friend had set him up and was being paid $155 to betray him.

Oddly, the Little Rock Police Department took no action at the time, and did not issue a warrant for Kevin's arrest until after Dr. Elders had made the now infamous statement some six months later. Surgeon General Elders made the statement on December 7, 1993 and eight days later a warrant was issued for Kevin's arrest.

The Trial

On July 18, 1994, Kevin was tried in Pulaski County Circuit Court by Judge John Plegge. That morning, before the trial, we had all gathered at Eric's house in Pine Bluff. After my morning walk I came back to Eric's house and told them I thought we needed to prepare ourselves for what would be rough going that day. Then the dam broke loose and Coach Elders could hold it in no longer. Oliver and Joycelyn both broke down and cried and went through the typical questioning of parents in that sort of circumstance, "what could we have done differently?" "Where did we go wrong?" I felt it was good for them to go through this process of dealing with the emotions of the moment, but I knew that they had been good parents. Sometimes it doesn't matter what kind of home, or whether a young person has the very best parents. The pressures and temptations are out there. What the family had to do at this point was to figure out how to go on from there; how to help Kevin get the help he needed to deal with his problems and straighten out his life.

Kevin testified that day at his trial before Judge Plegge that Walraven had blackmailed him into getting cocaine by threatening to go to the press about his (Kevin's) drug problem and personal life. Bowing to the pressure and thinking he could somehow prevent further problems for his mother in her work, he succumbed. The rest is a matter of history which has been widely publicized.

In court, Kevin's lawyer, Perlesta A. Hollingsworth, based his defense on entrapment. *The Arkansas Times* reported in the December 16, 1994 issues that

> *Hollingsworth claimed that Elders has no prior history of selling drugs; that he had repeatedly refused Walraven's request to do so, and that he had acquiesced to them only when Walraven threatened to tell the media about Kevin Elders' drug use and other allegations Walraven considered Kevin Elders would be threatened by. (Leveritt 14)*

In the end, Judge Plegge rejected the argument. He told Hollingsworth that he had not proven his charge of entrapment and he found Kevin guilty as charged. On August 29, 1994, Judge Plegge sentenced Kevin to ten years in prison.

As we exited the courthouse on the day of the trial a reporter asked Dr. Elders how she was doing. Her reply was that she was "as tough as an alligator." This statement made me think about an old story. Pretend for a moment that you are an alligator with a beautiful, valuable hide. One day your river homeland is invaded by hunters with spears. The hunters seem kind, but you are cautious and send the baby alligators out first. They pet them, but when you older alligators go out they attack and steal your hide — your heritage, the very essence of your being. They leave you to die, but they survive and grow stronger.

This little story may seem strange. It doesn't really make sense: the very thing that makes you who and what you are is the source of pain. It makes you confused and hate yourself and God for your hide — the very essence of your being. The question is, will you curse God for giving you such a valuable hide or give up and die? Or will you continue to be a proud alligator, just more cautious about approaching the hunters that invade your homeland?

I think Dr. Elders is an alligator who is proud of her hide. I think she knows the value of it and is thankful for it. It has enabled her to survive and grow stronger. I am confident that she will continue to be a proud, tough alligator.

Following the trial Kevin was released on bond pending his appeal. He continued to work for his family's real estate company while undergoing treatment for his drug addiction. He was ordered to submit to urine tests every two weeks. Throughout this ordeal his family has remained at his side. His mother, despite her busy schedule, finds time to be the leader of the pack when it comes to being there for Kevin.

Another blessing that we realized we had during this ordeal was that of some devoted, caring friends. One, in particular, was Sonya Hunt Gray. She now lives in Philadelphia, Pennsylvania and works for the Department of Health and Human Services out of Washington. She is an old friend of Kevin and our family. She heard about his troubles and his drug problem and took vacation time off her job to come and counsel and be with him for a couple of weeks. Our family will never forget her true friendship to Kevin when he needed her most. She and Kevin had taught a Sunday School class together at Hunter UMC when I was pastor there. The relationship that they built during this time prompted her to live out what she had taught in that class by coming for two weeks and going to group sessions at the Bridgeway treatment center with Kevin and giving support to her friend. Her visits and support helped Kevin when he needed it the most. This is a case of a person who was willing to lay down her life for a friend, which Jesus said was the greatest love of all (John 15:13). She had a great deal to do with helping Kevin to move along on the road to rehabilitation.

What Does It All Mean?

While my sister would probably disagree with this observation, it must be said. The story of Joycelyn Elders, including her son's arrest and conviction of selling drugs, holds a major part of the answer to the "riddle of the politics of drugs, race and sex."

The clues to this answer are clearly visible. The former Surgeon General is black, female, a medical doctor, outspoken and well-established by her own sweat and that of her loving husband, Oliver. She has something to say and she says it. She is not a politician, and she is not the type of black person who rises and learns to agree with whatever "the system" dictates just to survive herself. She is concerned for the masses. The woman has guts and, more than that, she has backbone. The sad truth is that too many in our society still are just not ready to accept this combination in any black person. They may not be readily accepting of it in any person. Joycelyn Elders dared to force us to deal with our own insecurities, biases, shame, ignorance and fears. She is rejected and rebuked mainly by the ultra right-wing conservatives of the country. Those who stand to lose the most if the masses can ever overcome their present conditions and circumstances. These groups are the ones who still insist on maintaining the status quo in America. Dr. Elders may not be the Surgeon General anymore, but America still has the same problems which she decries and is still wandering in the wilderness trying to find some resolution. The irony is one must first accept that there are problems before resolution can be found. This has been Dr. Elders' message, the one which has been rejected.

What we must try to understand, a part of the answer to the riddle, is why it has become more important in our society to take the side of what is politically expedient rather than taking the side of the truth. We are a people who seem to have become blinded by what is "politically expedient or correct." How did this happen? Of course, it should be easy to understand that when people insist on not really loving their neighbor as themselves, then there has to be someone who becomes the scapegoat.

When I think about what has happened here in our land, I look at my sister and the price she has paid, I wonder if she has not sacrificed herself to help us all understand many things about ourselves. Like it or not, she is one of several black leaders in America, and I, like so many others, wonder why it is that every time a strong black comes on the scene, that leader is somehow displaced. This has become the acceptable "political" reality. It is unfair, and no respecter of persons. It is a part of the answer to the riddle, a painful part which my sister knows only too well.

In spite of a system that has not always treated her fairly, my sister is fair. After learning of Kevin's arrest, she publicly stated that *"Kevin is my son, but he is not above the laws of the land."* Even though she was in a position of some political authority, she stayed within the bounds of the legal justice system.

This period has been a mixed experience for my sister and all her family. There has been joy and pain involved in the whole process, just as there is in being a parent. I know firsthand that Joycelyn has felt both the joy and pain of being a parent. She said, "*Kevin's drug addiction and trial "has helped me to see smell, taste, touch and feel the effects of the drug crisis in America. I have learned that being a mother is a lifetime commitment.*"

The Answer Becomes Clearer: Politics

As I have watched the events unfold regarding my sister's confirmation process, her tenure as Surgeon General and the arrest and conviction of her son, "the riddle of the politics of drugs, race and sex" seemed to become a little more distinct, if not clearer. For example, the proximity in time of the arrest of Kevin and the controversial statement by his mother seems more than coincidental. If one is tempted to accept the Little Rock Police Department's conclusion that there was no relationship between the two events, it is fair to say that the occurrence of the two, only eight days apart, is, at least, mystifying.

Another piece of the answer to the riddle, which is in itself puzzling, is found in the attack on Dr. Elders' family: the back social security taxes levied against her husband for the care of his invalid mother; the assessment of additional income taxes against me, and the unproved charges relating to property owned by the Elderses. Again, these things seem more than coincidental; they certainly could be politically motivated.

A third and difficult part of the answer to the riddle has to do with the lack of any action to investigate the charges allegedly made by Calvin Walraven that Herbert Jones, Jr. was the supplier of the illegal drugs. In a story reported by the *Arkansas Times* on December 16, 1994 it is stated that Chris Palmer, the Pulaski County prosecutor who put Walraven on the stand, insists Elders was not blackmailed or trapped into doing anything he hadn't already been doing. Palmer regrets that Elders never revealed the identity of his supplier, someone nicknamed "Tweet." Elders told police he believed he'd be killed if he told. But Palmer says that both society and Elders will be better off for his having been caught and sent to jail (Leveritt 15). Palmer is later quoted in the story as saying that *"the Kevin Elders bust was really a run-of-the-mill, simple case"* (Leveritt 15). The story says that Captain Sam Williams, head of the Little Rock Police Department's narcotics unit, agrees (Leveritt 15). According to the story Williams stated, *"I don't see any difference between this case and hundreds of other cases we make every year. As for the prominence of this individual's name (Elders, who is black), I can't do anything about that. We don't get to pick and choose who deals drugs"* (Leveritt 15).

The other fact pointed out in the story is that Herbert Jones, the alleged supplier initially implicated by Walraven has never been investigated. Jones happens to be white with a prominent name. When asked about it Williams said he had not been investigated and that *"he couldn't divulge precisely why,"* but he went on later to say that they simply "couldn't get to" Jones and that he "really didn't want to go into the circumstances behind that" (Leveritt 15). It seems there was a great deal of information about this part of the case which was not released. As to why Kevin Elders was arrested and charged. Williams did offer a reason, *"he was a dope dealer who an informant could deliver"* (Leveritt 15).

The fourth part of the answer to the riddle lies hidden in

the fact that the politicizing of race, drugs and sex is somewhat like the answer to the king's riddle given by his subject, "the only thing that does not change is change itself." It seems in our society the one thing that doesn't change is the politics of drugs, race and sex. To put it another way, the question is asked, "why does it appear that minorities and females who do not fit a certain mold are more harshly punished than are majority group males and females who run afoul of the law, or who otherwise offend or prick the conscience of the powers that be?" Also, why does the prominence of a person's name enter into this situation? This has been a long standing observation in our society. The politics seem to be clear and fairly strictly adhered to.

The Elderses' story demonstrates that up through the Twentieth Century not much has changed. The riddle of the politics of drugs, race and sex is still a problem to be solved in America. This problem is evidenced in one of the unspoken tragedies of this case, that is the fact that a young person used as an informant to set up others obviously became so saddened and overwhelmed by all the dealings surrounding him that he could not go on facing it anymore. Unfortunately, the week following the trial, he shot and killed himself. And Kevin Elders, facing time in prison, still awaits the judicial process to run its course for him. Two young lives have been permanently affected by this situation. Such tragedies and waste of human life are good reasons for us to become serious about solving the riddle of politics, drugs, race and sex in America.

They Called Him 'Mr. Witt'

The reality of politics is powerful in our country. Another example of this sort of political witch-hunting is the Whitewater matter that has plagued Arkansas for some time now. Whitewater is a conspiracy to destroy the political and economic base in Arkansas. It is not just about President Clinton. It is about what a Northern Wall Street economic network and powerful mid-West and Northern political tier call the greatest mistake to happen in this country since Wal-Mart. Wal-Mart discount stores are still considered to be a mistake that never should have happened according to powerful Northern, Mid-Western and Northwestern business families. These groups are now spreading propaganda by sending large donations to religious T.V. evangelists to destroy the moral character of anyone that they see as a political threat from Arkansas. They have used this network to try and destroy Dr. Elders, the present Governor and are determined to bring down President Clinton, because they feel a little state like Arkansas has no right to such a powerful political and economic base. I understand the Whitewater investigators have now accused Governor Tucker of falsifying his loan request to the Old Testament patriarch, Methuselah, who died about five thousand years ago. Where does it all end? These business family cartels will stop at nothing less than destroying the whole economic and political infra-structure of the state. The bottom line is that over the past thirty years the Stephens family, who owns one of the largest off-Wall Street brokerage firms, with advice from one of the most powerful congressmen and political consultants on tax laws this nation ever had, Wilber Mills (who maintained his power until his bout with Fanny Fox and downfall from addiction to alcohol) was able to set up an economic oasis in one of the least expected places in the country, Little Rock. While the whole country was so focused and paralyzed on what was happening at Central High School, and President Eisenhower was selecting Little Rock as the place to test the Southern resolve to fight school integration, the Stephens family, under the leadership of the late Witt Stephens, economic and political guru, was quietly going about their business, setting and building up one of the most powerful family economic bases in the country. This family has quietly gone about its business and helped to make and create more millionaires in Arkansas over the last thirty years than any other family owned empire in the world. It would not have been possible for the growth and development of businesses like Dillard's, Wal-Mart, J.B. Hunt Trucking, Tyson Chicken, TCBY and a whole list of other Arkansas family businesses without the help and backing of the Stephens family. This family has not only been successful in business ventures, but it has been successful in backing and supporting the right political candidates, until the untimely death of the family business and political guru, who in Arkansas was known until his death as "Mr. Witt." Arkansas could never have grown and groomed an American president without the powerful network of the Stephens family empire.

Now the whole purpose of the Whitewater investigation is to paralyze the political and business dealings in Arkansas the same way it has destroyed the public education in the state by keeping the state education system in hock to a federal court judge for over thirty years. This court battle has almost destroyed the Little Rock School District to the point that it cannot keep a school superintendent, it cannot keep many students, nor teachers. The same paradigm is now being set up by the Whitewater investigation. Once the camel (the federal government) sticks its nose under the tent in a small state like Arkansas, you can bet your last dollar that the camel will slowly work to get his tail inside the tent as well. And when that happens, no citizens in the state are safe. The federal government, still under control of Northern businesses and political bosses are only using the Whitewater investigation in Arkansas in the same way it used Central High School to try and destroy public education in the state. I hope I am around long enough to say about the Whitewater investigation the same thing many black and white citizens are saying now about the federal government sending troops to straighten out the Little Rock School District, "I told you so."

The answer to the riddle of the political games of our nation is that we have sat by for too long and allowed politicians to run amuck and trample many good people. Such political debacles, as the Savings and Loan scandal are proof that politicians are not primarily concerned about the best interest of the whole country, they are primarily concerned about the best interests of the rich and powerful. Likewise, they are against anyone who tries to stand for the best interests of the common folk, the poor and the powerless. This is why Dr. Elders was ousted, and it is why the Whitewater ordeal has been allowed to be blown so out of proportion. The "bear" has gone wild and is trying to eat up everyone who tries to protect those who are weaker.

Chapter Seventeen

THE PARADIGM OF SEX, RACE AND SACRIFICE

Age Old Paradigm

We know all too well how ancient men felt about women, and the role of women in ancient society; we know very little about how those women felt about themselves. There are significant parallels, however, between ancient and modern prejudice and it is safe to assume that the self-image of women fostered by patriarchal society is essentially the same in all centuries. *"Prejudice is not something which takes place on the periphery of man, as though he had acquired a stain upon the garments of personality by brushing up against the social order; it has its locus rather in the deep interior of man's being"* (Haselden 78). Women in general, and Black and other ethnic women in particular, have always been socially approved victims of prejudice and discrimination.

Prejudice has always been a necessary narcotic for humanity. History reflects a clear record to prove this.

> *Every group has another group upon which it projects all that is by its standards odious and in which, by contrast, it sees its own glorification reflected. The Jews had the Gentiles; the Greeks had Barbarians; the Romans had non-Romans; the Crusaders had their infidels; the Fifteenth Century Roman Catholics had their heathens; the English had the Irish; the Lutherans had the Anabaptists; the Nazis had the non-Aryans. (Graham 211)*

The subjugation of women by men in all aspects of society is part and parcel of this sort of discrimination and has been a common practice in almost all cultures.

Contempt for women is not an accident; it is a by-product of culture. The culture is founded on it. It is the essential core; without it, the culture would fall apart. No matter what we say about women's rights, and how much progress we have made, we still have not reached an era of post-feminist equality. This is evidenced by the ways that women's advocacy groups are viewed in our society. When the time comes when men are willing to admit they are no longer the dominant force in our society, even though they are in the minority numerically, and form advocacy groups for themselves then some sort of equilibrium will have been achieved. But as long as women's groups, like the National Organization of Women, etc., are disparaged by a patriarchal controlled culture, then women are not yet equal.

Marilyn French catalogs several examples of the effect the patriarchy has on women:

> *The harm done to women in the name of fundamentalist religions and cultural customs, including the genital mutilation of women in Africa, bride burning in India, and female infanticide in China, instances of sexual discrimination and harassment in government and business, and rape and domestic violence, including incest, batter and murder....* (Graham 211)

This inherent sexism affects all women, but it is particularly harsh for those women who dare to step into the public realm. I would be hard pressed to name a single woman of public note in our society who has not fallen under the ridicule of the patriarchy. From the earliest times in the history of America women who have asserted themselves and their gifts have been criticized and controlled by patriarchal society. For instance, early women writers had to have a male "sponsor" to vouch for the worth of their literary works before they could be published and often these men profited financially from the women's work while the women themselves received very little financial reward for their work. The women who stepped forward to champion the abolition, temperance and suffrage movements were ridiculed. In more modern times women who have ventured beyond the careers long deemed "acceptable" for women (e.g. teachers, nurses, secretaries) have been ridiculed and rejected. Certainly I can attest to the patriarchal attitude of the church as I have watched clergywomen struggle for acceptance in the church and have seen many of them become discouraged and give up. We have witnessed in the last three years a glut of sexist insults hurled at women political leaders, and have seen and heard especially vitriolic words spoken about Hillary Rodham Clinton who has not exactly fit the role traditionally deemed "acceptable" for a First Lady. And of course, I cannot help but feel that the treatment my sister received was partially due to the fact that she is a woman, and worse still, a Black woman. Dr. Elders has said she feels that "Black women must stand up and speak out against prejudice and sexism and not allow themselves to be victimized by males who will steal their purity for selfish gratification." She knows from experience that this is not any easy thing to do, but she has pressed on out of her personal assurance that the differences of sex, and race, are not intrinsic, but are evils created by society. She knows all too painfully well the price exacted from one who dares to live out a truly inclusive life in an exclusive world.

Hit Her Where She's Vulnerable

Racism exacerbated by prejudice and sexism and right-wing religious politics made every effort to destroy Dr. Elders first as a person, second as a woman—and an outspoken woman at that— and third as a Black American. Only after these groups could not destroy her on these fronts did they start to dig around into the affairs of her family members; if they could not do her in directly, perhaps they could reach her where a woman is most vulnerable, her family.

In today's still-patriarchal society, as in ancient times, a wife's self-worth and social status often pivot around her husband. Therefore, when traditional methods failed to derail Dr. Elders' confirmation as U.S. Surgeon General, right-wing religious and conservative political groups conspired to destroy her by trying socially and economically to destroy the reputation of her husband. Thus Dr. Elders' reputation was called into question, not because she was not qualified professionally, but because her husband did not let her become involved in his family's business decisions. Never mind the stark fact is that such areas are off-limits to in-laws who do not want to become outlaws! As in ancient times, Dr. Elders' qualifications were judged on her husband's failure to pay Social Security taxes on a home health care worker who took care of his ailing ninety-five year old mother. Her husband, who is a socially prominent, successful basketball coach, was humiliated and characterized as irresponsible for trying to help his parents through a sickness and death, as most children will do for their sick parents. In his case, he did not think about all the business aspects of bringing his mother home to live with him. Because of this mistake, the family was exploited, persecuted and socially castrated. For many families, such an ordeal would have caused domestic differences, for the Elders family it was an occasion for them to come closer together.

"The More Things Change..."

The other area where our society has not changed much in the last 150 years is in the area of racial prejudice. Even this many years this side of the Civil War and almost four decades passed the Civil Rights battles, we still are battling each other on racial grounds. In Arkansas we still battle school desegregation issues. In the town where I live during this writing we have recently witnessed a battle on the city government level on racial issues. In the last several years we have witnessed numerous racially motivated incidents, like the Rodney King ordeal in Los Angeles. And, while I would like to believe it is not true, many African Americans believe that the Senate's refusal to confirm Dr. Henry Foster as Dr. Elders' successor for Surgeon General is racially motivated. It seems that they will not settle for having three ethnics in succession in the office. It seems that we are no closer to racial harmony than we are to gender equality.

Gunnar Myrdal characterized the arena of conflict long ago when he said: "*The democracy we profess and the democracy we practice when it comes to Black women is a problem of the heart. . . The American Negro problem is a problem in the heart of Americans*" (xlvii). In America, under the tutelage of largely Christian white-male-dominated society, "*race prejudice is learned; religious bigotry is learned; social snobbery is learned; but they can be learned only because they have an apt and eager pupil in the inherently prideful and instinctively prejudiced will of [humans]*" (Haselden 80). What can be learned, of course, can be changed. A small step toward making such change came recently when the Southern Baptist Convention issued their apology for their racist past. I was surprised and pleased to hear of their apology to African Americans. I was also shocked by it in the midst of the conservative Republican political climate rampant today I did not expect this sort of an act of repentance. The political and social atmosphere today does not seem to me to be one inclined toward apologies from conservatives, yet the Southern Baptists stood up and did so. This simply proves the old saying, "God works in mysterious ways, His wonders to perform." Perhaps there is some hope that we can learn different behaviors. But it will take more than simple apologies to right the centuries of oppression. It will take a change in the power structure as well.

Racism has been defined as "prejudice plus power." When prejudices, bigoted ideas are coupled with power then the opportunity for oppression of one group by another exists. We must work together to learn to share power, rather than trying to gain more power and hoard it. Only when we can learn to do this can we make a dent in racism, and sexism, too, for that matter.

Another case in point is the debate currently being waged around Affirmative Action. To me, this is more a moral issue than a political issue. My problem with the current debate centers around the silence of the church on this issue. The legislation passed in the last few decades was certainly not passed out of the goodness of politicians' hearts. Rather, the Civil Rights movement created a climate where a Southerner, Lyndon Johnson (in my opinion the best President since Lincoln), got legislation through providing for affirmative action programs. So, this issue has never been a purely political one. It has always been centered in the moral justice of God. It serves to highlight the sin of racism, which is a sin not against a particular race of people, but is a sin against God who created all people. As the Psalmist says "*against thee, thee only have I sinned...*" (Psalm 51:4 KJV) So issues like affirmative action, which has at its core issue like racial justice, will not be solved in Washington; they will be solved in churches, temples, mosques and other places of worship.

Painful Lessons

Dr. Elders certainly learned about racism through firsthand experience, but yet, she steadfastly refuses to join in dwelling on this painful reality. She has been able to bridge over the scars of the past and to overcome the painful past of racism we have experienced. In the South black people were treated very badly. We all know the stories of segregated schools, lunch counters, washrooms, drinking fountains, seating in public places and transportation. I recall and puzzle over now, for instance, that when Joycelyn and I were growing up our parents never discussed why the girls never had any baby dolls as Christmas presents, like other little girls. Instead, some black parents bought teddy bears for their children for Christmas. Teddy bears were certainly fashionable in the black community at that time. Parents could not give their children a lot at Christmas, but for their second Christmas most children received a teddy bear. The children played with them to fill up the empty times in their lives. A teddy bear could be cuddled at night in bed and was also nurturing and comforting to a child. My grandmother had recommended that our parents buy one for Joycelyn. She took it with her everywhere. In the winter she would cuddle up in bed with it; it was a magical warmth when there was no heat in the room. Whenever she could not get her way, she would find comfort in talking to her teddy bear. The teddy bear met a special need for rural black children. Now I am now not sure whether the black parents were making a statement against racism, because there were no Black baby dolls in rural Southwest Arkansas, or whether they were simply buying teddy bears for children to sleep with in the cold rooms of the shotgun shacks we all lived in. I don't know why, but at this point I am afraid to ask. That will have to be the third question I will ask my parents in heaven.

But even in the face of the painful racist realities of our lives, Joycelyn always seemed to live beyond them. She never accepted the segregated reality of the South. The best example of Joycelyn's beliefs is the incident alluded to in earlier chapters of this book. It happened at the Elberta Drive-In Theatre in Nashville, Arkansas. Joycelyn had taken us to the movies to see *Old Yeller*. The film was made by Walt Disney in the 1950's about a poor Texas family in the 1860's, and a wonderful old dog, "Old Yeller." It was a movie that paralleled so much of what life was like for us growing up as sharecroppers in Southwest Arkansas. However, the warmth and love of this memorable movie has also left in my memory the racial incident that almost caused us to miss seeing the film. It all began after my sister had purchased the tickets for herself, my two younger sisters and me. We were told to park, as usual, in the back section reserved for the "Coloreds." Joycelyn, however, refused at first to park all the way back in the "Colored Section," and instead parked near the last row reserved for whites. After she parked an attendant came and asked her "what she thought she was doing?" "You know you can't park here." "That's the rule." I was afraid and puzzled. I could see that Joycelyn was hurt and angry, the angriest I had ever seen her. She didn't understand why, when she had paid for her tickets the same as everyone else, that she should be forced to park in the back. I wondered what on earth they had done to her mind in Little Rock at Philander Smith College. I feared for our safety, and even our lives when Joycelyn told the attendant that she would leave before she would move all the way back in the "Colored Section." By this time we had begun to cry, partly out of fear, and perhaps largely because we didn't want to miss the movie because of what I then thought of as my sister's insane stubbornness. We cried and begged and finally Joycelyn gave in and moved back a couple of rows to the "Colored Section," where she grudgingly stayed to see the movie.

When I think back on this incident, I am pained by the cruel realities of racial prejudice that were a part of our growing up. At the same time, I am proud to have a sister like Joycelyn who has never believed that discrimination was right on any level, for any reason. She has always stood up for what she knew to be right. It is her uncompromising stance for the right which has carried her as far as she has gone, and which has also caused problems for her along the way. But she has been willing to pay the price required in order to maintain a stand for the right. Joycelyn, unlike her brother who would, at the time, have watched *Old Yeller* though a peep-hole in the back of the theater, refused to compromise her belief that it was wrong to have a double standard for black and white, rich and poor, then and it is wrong now.

Taking a Stand

I, unfortunately, have not always been as brave about taking a stand as Joycelyn. It has taken years of retrospection for me to learn the importance of standing for what is right, something that Joycelyn has long done. I remember the time in 1962 while I was in the Army stationed in North Carolina with the 82nd Airborne. General Walker had gone to Oxford, Mississippi to the University of Mississippi to keep the first black student, James Meredith, from enrolling there. The 82nd Airborne was called in to help keep order. We were flown to an Airbase just outside Jackson. Word came to us that the crowds were throwing rocks at the black troops and so the decision had been made to pull out all black troops and so we would not be going to Ole Miss. At the time I was 18 years old and was happy not to have to go and be involved in the rioting. My Sergeant, however, felt differently. Sgt. Hightower, a twenty year career Army man, was mad that we were not going to be allowed to go. He said that he was a soldier and that his job was to go deal with conflict. He didn't want to stay away simply because we were black. Myself, I was still relieved. I was happy to sleep safely in my pup tent. I was glad not to be sent to the front lines of the conflict to deal with the enemy — the enemy which is anything that separates us, even people of our own country or our own household. Now I know that it was like sleeping through a great revolution. Now I have the 20-20 vision of hindsight. I know that there are times when we simply must take a stand and we must risk whatever is necessary to make that stand. I hope that we will not have to wait another 33 years to realize that some things are so dear that, when you are called to go, are worth fighting and dying for.

Chapter Eighteen

LIBERTY DENIED

*...One nation under God, indivisible,
with Liberty and Justice for All.*

<u>The Day Dr. Elders was Fired</u>

I had been out that day to pick up my wife, Valarie, at the airport, after which we went to Park Plaza Mall in Little Rock to do some Christmas shopping. We returned home that evening, December 9, 1994, about 5:30 p.m. As I drove into the driveway and got out of the car, I could hear the phone ringing. Like most people, I felt the sense of urgency to find the keys and get into the house before it stopped. And, this particular time, I almost sensed a distress in the way the phone rang. It kept ringing until I got into the house and answered it.

The voice on the other end of the line said, "Have you heard what happened to your sister?" There was a long pause as I thought about all the things that could have happened. After a moment the caller said, "Bill Clinton fired your sister!" With a sigh of relief I said, "Well, she can come home now that her time in Washington has expired." The caller went on to tell me what he thought of the President for having bowed to pressure in firing her. I stopped him and said, "Doctor, the President did Joycelyn a favor; after the November elections Washington, including the President, is under a new management." As we spoke my thoughts were churning. I told him that I believed that rather than compromise her principles, or bow to political pressure and become just another figurehead Surgeon General, Dr. Elders should come home while she still had her faith in what I call the

American birthright—liberty. I compared her to Patrick Henry when it comes to Liberty. She'd choose to die rather than have her liberty denied. In reply the caller spoke words of courage, and affirmation and shared how much he appreciated and respected what Dr. Elders did as Surgeon General. I thanked him for all his support and we ended the phone conversation.

I shared with Valarie what had happened and we switched on the television to watch the evening news. Sure enough, the headline on all three networks was that the President had fired the Surgeon General for having used the "M" word while speaking at the United Nations on World AIDS Day.

Immediately I began trying to reach my sister at her home in Bethesda, Maryland. I finally got her husband on the phone. We talked for a moment and he said "here is your sister." When she got to the phone I said, "Joycelyn, you may not see or understand it now, but I believe this has happened for the best." I told her that "every cloud has a silver lining" and that "all things work together for good when you love the Lord" (Romans 8:28 NEB). I went on to ask, "Now, what can I do to help you and Oliver move back home?" The conversation ended on a good note with Joycelyn saying, "Thanks, Chess, I needed that call and support."

The next morning I called Joycelyn again to check on how they were doing and found they were still in the process of reviewing their options. Oliver still had his job with the U.S. Department of Education in Washington and Joycelyn was to discuss with someone in the Department of Health and Human Services a job they were offering her in the National Health Core. Needless to say, that tree bore no fruit.

After thinking about the opportunities in Washington, Oliver told Joycelyn that he had come there with her for her to assume the position of Surgeon General and, now that the time was up, he was ready to return to Arkansas. Meanwhile, Dr. Harry Ward, Chancellor at the University of Arkansas School of Medical Sciences had called and offered Joycelyn her old job at Children's Hospital, where she was a tenured professor.

In a later phone conversation, Joycelyn told me of Dr. Ward's offer. I could hear a familiar ring of delight in her voice. At that point, I knew she would also weather this storm because she had come to realize that it is more important to do the job as Surgeon General than to have the job. Joycelyn has always been more concerned about truth than about politics. Only when one knows the truth can that person interpret the intent behind the political storm that called for Dr. Elders' resignation.

Now that I felt a calming of the storm I wanted to know "from the horse's mouth" exactly what she had said. I wanted to know if she thought she might have been better off to sidestep the question. Of course, I was very quickly put in my place. She let me know that she understood the politics of sidestepping controversial issues, but when it comes to being a doctor and public official, she did not believe the people desire, or deserve, hypocrisy, political or otherwise. She explained that even when the facts are distasteful, they should be dealt with forthrightly and honestly by doctors, scientists and, especially, the Surgeon General because of the nature of that position. "You see, Chester," she said, "*masturbation, or the 'm' word, is part of human sexuality whether we like it or not. Therefore, I believe where it is appropriate, the topic should be a part of our basic education process. As I have said so many times before, we have tried ignorance for a long, long time; why not try education?*"

Sensing that she was willing to talk for a while, I asked her, "Joycelyn, what did you really say?" In reply, she wasted no time in getting right to the heart of her statement which she recalled as this, "*...I think that it (masturbation) is something that is part of human sexuality and it is part of something that perhaps should be taught. But we've not even taught our children the very basics. I feel that we have tried ignorance for a very long time, and it's time to try education....*" After hearing the statement from Joycelyn herself, I was somewhat mystified and I was trying to be objective about the matter. I had started to doubt my understanding of the word and how it fit into the various forms of sexual behavior, so I set out to bone up on the subject.

First, I reviewed the dictionary definition. Then I cross referenced the term under the subtopic of "exploring sexuality" in the "Physical Intimacy" chapter of an old college textbook by Ernest J. Green, *Personal Relationships, An Approach to Marriage and Family*. While I will not attempt to give a review of that part of the work, the material was informative, it proved that Joycelyn was correct in what she said. It also gave me added insight into the political commotion the statement prompted.

Why? What Evil has She Done?

Most people realize by now that in a technical sense, Dr. Elders, the first African American and second woman in the history of the United States to serve as Surgeon General, was summarily fired by President Clinton. The $64,000 question is, "for what reason, or reasons, was she fired?" Isn't it curious that in all the press coverage that followed the firing, no one in the White House, or elsewhere, has yet to face the nation and state in clear, unambiguous language the specific act, or acts, Elders is accused of having committed. Yet it was for these unspecified reasons that she was "asked to resign," or be fired. In fact, the position taken by the White House has been more or less a "no comment" attitude. So, the question is, "What is Elders' crime?" Why was she punished without any semblance of due process?

It has been suggested that perhaps hers is what some observers call "speech crimes." Perhaps there is some merit to their argument. Others suggest that President Clinton simply weighed his political goods and buckled under the weight of the political pressure of the Republicans, religious right and conservatives. He made a hasty decision to sacrifice Elders, an outspoken African-American, woman doctor who had perhaps become too much of a thorn in the side of Clinton's administration because she resisted being muzzled as a public official.

While there are many who agree that the firing only validates the feeling that African Americans and women are taken for granted by the Clinton Administration, there are those of us who would like to believe that this is not the case. However, we have only the record to look to for explanations.

As for Elders, since no real public explanation of her firing has been offered by the Clinton Administration, the public is left to assume that the firing resulted from Dr. Elders remarks made in New York after a speech at the United Nations on World AIDS Day, December 1, 1994. It is a fact that she was fired on December 9, 1994, only eight days later.

The censured remark was given when Dr. Elders took a question from Dr. Clark, a psychologist and AIDS Conference Panel Member. The discussion was as follows

> *Dr. Clark: It seems to me that the campaign against AIDS has already destroyed many taboos about discus-*

sion of sex in public. It seems to me that there still remains, however, a taboo against discussion about masturbation, and, please forgive me for trying to do my tiny bit by announcing that I masturbate, and I do want to ask you, what do you think are the prospects of a more explicit discussion and promotion of masturbation?

Dr. Elders: Dr. Clark, I think you already know that I am a very strong advocate of a comprehensive health education program, if you will, starting at a very early age. I feel that it should be age-appropriate, it should be complete, and we need to teach our children all of the things that they need to know. And we know that many of our parents have difficulties teaching certain things, and for that reason, to make sure that all of our children are more informed, I've always felt that we should, you know, that we should make it a part of our school. I feel it's the only institution that we have where all of the children go, and presently in our schools, it is very incomplete; it's very petty, and only a few of our schools have a comprehensive program. To address your specific question in regard to masturbation, I think it is something that is a part of human sexuality, and it is a part of something that perhaps should be taught. We've not even taught our children the very basics, and I feel that we have tried ignorance for a very long time, and it's time we try education.

For this statement, the President asked Dr. Elders to resign. In essence, what she said was that masturbation should be taught as being a normal part of human sexuality, not that masturbation should be taught to non-age-appropriate children, or to replace or avoid sexual relations with a partner. The literature on the subject supports Dr. Elders' position.

In some cultures, the subject is more widely discussed

than in others. Obviously, it is still a taboo topic in certain places in America. However, that does not erase the fact that it is a part of human sexuality or that it is one of the ways in which sexual behavior can be learned. Again, a search of the literature supports this position. In *Personal Relationships, An Approach to Marriage and Family,* Ernest J. Green includes the following information:

> *Masturbation is one of the best means we have of learning about our bodies about sex directly – without fear, hesitancy, guilt, or shyness. Since all of the genital areas is an erogenous zone, through masturbation one can discover the specific areas of greatest sensitivity and the means and mechanisms of sexual responsiveness (Eisner).*
>
> *In contrast to this growing contemporary appraisal of masturbation is the list of symptoms and ailments once attributed to the practice (Katchadourian and Lunde). Included are insanity, epilepsy, asthma, hallucinations, and acne. There is also a curious and tragic history of threats and punishments used to curtail masturbation (or cure its alleged symptoms), including removal of the clitoris. The unfortunate aspect for us today is that the topic of masturbation is still shadowed by prejudice, misinformation, and guilt. If given its proper evaluation, however, it may be that the only detrimental aspect of masturbation is psychological and social one – especially, the continual use of masturbation and masturbatory fantasies as a substitute for, or way of avoiding sexual exploration with another human being. (82)*

Many people, even small children, before they reach their teenage years, will have experienced masturbation. However, very few will ever admit to, or talk about it. Most young people are not taught at home or school concerning the topic, and, as a result, many go around feeling guilty and negative about themselves.

In other instances, most adults are more aware of the fact that masturbation has been used as a method of relieving sexual tension. Others may choose to engage in appropriate flesh-based relations instead. Still others may choose celibacy as an alternative. It is a tough debate.

African Americans: Still in Search of Freedom of Speech

Both Joycelyn Elders and C. Everett Koop served as United States Surgeon General. Both took some rather controversial stands on issues. However, there are major differences in the two. Koop is white, male and a conservative. Elders is African American, female and a pragmatist.

Mary Frances Berry, a U.S. Civil Rights Commissioner and the Geraldine R. Segal Professor of American Social Thought and History at the University of Pennsylvania does a wonderful job of analyzing the differences in Koop and Elders. She is quoted in an article in the December 19, 1994 issue of *Black Issues in Higher Education* by Mary Christine Phillips titled, "Taken for Granted Again":

> *... This is not the first time that a Surgeon General has talked about masturbation. What Elders didn't realize was that she could not do what former Surgeon General C. Everett Koop did. She is a Black woman and he is a white man. He said a lot of the same things she is saying. He talked about masturbation, he talked about AIDS and made the same recommendations,' Berry says. 'There is a booklet he put out about AIDS and sex education, and masturbation was part of it. But the fact is he was conservative, and although he said controversial things, he is a white man. It is a different ball game for her [Elders] as a black woman.... (28-29)*

Like Berry, many people may wonder if Elders just failed

to recognize the difference. I suspect that she did recognize the difference, but chose not to give credence to the differences because her philosophy of life has always been centered around the belief that no one should be limited by race, creed, color, place of birth or gender, but only by the size of their hopes and dreams. Dr. Elders' vision has always been focused beyond the day-to-day troubles of race, creed and color to the heights of hope. She has never been one to see color as a handicap. However, I often reminded her that because of our history in America there are things a black person, and a black woman in particular, still can't say.

As I pondered the question of the difference between a white male and Black female Surgeon General's authority and power, my mind drifted back to the incident with Joycelyn at the movie Old Yeller. In her own way she has always fought the battle and resisted unequal treatment of minorities and women. However, with her it is not always a conscious thing, it is just a part of her nature to believe that if the Constitution says something then that is the way it is for all people. Likewise, she believes that all God's people have the same God-given right to be free. She does not accept the idea that people should be judged and treated according to the color of their skin or their sex. In whatever she does, she acts according to her belief and does not usually compromise for political reasons. Joycelyn has always been able to put good sense above good politics. Thus, she may have assumed that she could speak freely as a medical doctor from the "bully pulpit" of the Surgeon General's office. What is wrong with that picture? Koop was allowed to do so. Why not Elders?

The President's move to silence Elders may have come as a surprise to her since she knew that he was aware that she has been frank in her discussions of health issues for years. That piece of the puzzle does not fit. Yet, it is clear from the number of times the Administration moved to publicly distance itself from her statements that there was not a meeting of the minds. Whether this represented a lack of teamwork, or just another way of eventually building a case to topple and silence her, who knows?

It is clear that Elders felt strongly about the issues for which she went out on a limb, and she refused to be silenced. What else are we to assume? She is most certainly an intelligent woman. And, having been an administrator herself, she probably did realize that if she continued to exercise such free and forthright speech she would be fired. Knowing my sister, she chose to stand up for open discussion of the issues over the job. That is vintage Joycelyn Elders.

In retrospect, we must wonder if the same sinister relationship was at work between the failure to appoint Black women such as Lani Guinier, Johnnetta Cole and the firing of Joycelyn Elders. What is it that these Black women have in common? What is it about them that seems to turn off conservative? All three women are very well educated, intelligent, accomplished in their fields, credentialed and strong in their personalities. What is it that causes these Black women to be denied opportunities for which they qualify and have earned the privilege? Sometimes blacks feel there is still an ethnic cleansing at work in Washington politics seeking to limit the power of minorities, and a gender cleansing seeking to limit women. With all due respect to the Black women who remain in the Administration, we do have to ask who and where they are? With Elders removal how many visible Black women are left in the Administration? There is Hazel O'Leary in the Cabinet, but the others are scarce. It is also noteworthy that there is not a single black woman on the Supreme Court, though there has certainly been ample opportunity to appoint one, and there is only one woman in the Senate, Carol Moseley-Braun from Illinois, who strongly supported Joycelyn and is herself very strong and outspoken.

The firing of Dr. Elders is most troubling for two major reasons. First, throughout her stint as Surgeon General, it was apparent from the treatment she received by certain groups and administration officials that the practice of token appointments for minorities and women continues in America. They might be appointed, but they are to be seen and not heard. The old saying holds, "the more things change, the more they stay the same." It is a practice long recognized and scorned by certain minority groups and women's advocacy proponents. It is a negative practice that should be brought out in the open and exposed to honest discussion and resolution. Another way to help alleviate the problem is for more women and minority group representatives to be willing to take a firm and unpopular stand, as Dr. Elders did. And yes, perhaps even to be fired in order to expose the racist and sexist pattern of discrimination and denial of liberty.

A second reason why the firing of Dr. Elders is so troubling is that it possibly holds serious implications as it relates to the right of public officials to exercise freedom of speech in the performance of the duties. Except where free speech by public officials falls within the limitations determined by the U.S. Supreme Court, we believe public officials must be free to speak without fear of reprisal. We must guarantee such free speech whether we agree with them or resent their presence and personalities. This is one of the basic rights our country is founded on, and one we hear claimed by all sorts of extremist groups. If it applies to extremist groups and hate groups, shouldn't it also apply to public officials who are trying to responsibly do their jobs? Jackie Robinson, who integrated major league baseball by signing with the Brooklyn Dodgers in

1947, was once described somewhere as "a man with a chip on his shoulder" because of his outspokenness late in his career. People wanted him to be less outspoken. Sports legend attributes Robinson as saying, "I just could not do that. It would be like taking a third strike without attempting to hit the ball." Dr. Elders, likewise, could not simply be silent in order to be politically correct. Senator Moseley-Braun said of Dr. Elders during debate on the Senate floor,

> ...Dr. Elders has always spoken the truth; has always told it as she saw it. She has spoken her mind, spoken truthfully and honestly to the issues and concerns of the American people with regard to their public health. She has talked about her concern for children, sometimes in controversial context, but she has talked about her concern for children with a consistent truth that rings so loudly it is inescapable to any person who has reviewed her work and followed her discussion of the issues over time. (U.S. Cong. Joint Committee on Printing S10987-8)

Many have not liked Dr. Elders' straight-forward presentation of the truth, many have sought to misinterpret it, but the truth remains for any who would hear it.

The surprise in the firing of Dr. Elders is the fact that the President knuckled under and succumbed to pure political pressure fraught with racism and sexism designed to silence her. Politics, not policy, were the reason for her firing and it seems that all politics are influenced by self-interest. The act could be interpreted as an example for anybody else who dares to be heard and isn't a white male. We have seen similar indictments in the sinister attacks leveled against such figures as Ron Brown, Mike Espy, Henry Cisneros and Dr. Henry Foster, President Clinton's choice as the successor for Dr. Elders.

While I agree with my friend J. M. Lawson, (See letter at the end of this chapter) still, in the face of the situation as it stands today, I believe that President Clinton is a good man. The regret is that he let himself fall prey to such sinister pressure as he did. The real tragedy of our political system is that officials feel they must give in to such pressure in order to be elected and re-elected. However, the President is forgiven for taking actions in effort to preserve his political position, and he is still loved by our family. To this day Joycelyn has never said one negative word about the President. She still feels that he will go down in history as being a great two-term President. I personally, even as a minister, sometimes find it hard to believe how much unconditional love that my sister has for the President. It is only human to feel some measure of resentment in this sort of situation, but not Joycelyn. She still loves her President and supports him fully, and so do I. Joycelyn will always be grateful to President Clinton for inviting her to the "dance" as Surgeon General in his administration. Joycelyn says, "you should never forget who invited you to the dance." And, unfortunately, when one gets involved in politics it is important to remember that there are no permanent dance partners, someone or something else may cut-in. Politics are not always pleasant and good men like President Clinton sometimes have to bow to political pressure in order to preserve their interests in the long term, this is the unfortunate reality of the dance of politics—sometimes someone taps you on the shoulder and forces you and your partner apart. We pray that as he continues his political dance in Washington President Clinton will be able to muster the strength he will surely need to allow the power of the Lord to work through him as he helps to "insure justice, and domestic tranquillity, provide for the common defense, promote the general welfare and the blessings of life, liberty and the pursuit of happiness for all of us.

(Letter from J.M.Lawson, Jr, Pastor Holman United Methodist Church, Los Angeles, California, to the President of the United States)

December 20, 1994

The President
The White House
1600 Pennsylvania Avenue, NW
Washington, DC 20500

Dear Mr. President:

I want you to know that in 1996, you will not have my support for re-election. It will be the first time as an adult that I will not be voting for the democratic candidate fo President. I will not vote for the Republican, of course, since they offer nothing but horror for millions of people if not for the world.

WHY?

1. You did what I suspected you would do. You asked for the resignation of Dr. Joceyln Elders, one of the best things you have in your favor. You fired her because of the animosity of your Chief of Staff and the so called right wing conservative pressures.

2. In firing her you "trashed" your third African American woman of excellent work, experiences, talent, intelligence, character and grace. Even before you assumed office, you permitted that to happen with Dr. Johnetta Coles, President of Spellman College who you considered for appointment. You ran away from Lani Grenier (after telling yourself lies about her work). Three times, my dear Friend, you have not had the character or courage to simply fulfill the ethical dimensions of friendship all because of the "political" game you are playing ... a game which will force you to be a one term President.

3. Generally, you have turned your back on the multi-faceted coalition which elected you. We voted for you because you called for a 50 billion a year "re-investment in

American", jobs, universal health care, education, to end homelessness, etc. Because of your campaign speeches, which also criticized the callousness of Presidnet Bush and his public policies, you put together a genuine coalition and won. Since then you have simply gone over and adopted the Bush Administration budget, military program, economic program and NAFTA.

You are a far better man than you have been President. You can still restore the earlier vision you had for this country. Mark my word: you can still be re-elected in 1996, if that is what you want.

Holman is a congregation that prays for your family and you almost weekly. In the Communion Service I administer each Friday morning, we mention you by name. But you are not being the President you were called to be or the President the scriptures propose.

If not now, when?

SHALOM in this season and beyond.

J.M. Lawson, Jr.
Pastor

CONVICTIONS

When you are dancing with a bear,
You can't get tired and sit down;
You must wait until the bear gets tired,
Then you sit down.

Her message often is much more explosive than her laugh. She brought with her to the office of Surgeon General very strong convictions. None of them was about trying to be a part of the Washington political or social scenes. M. Joycelyn Elders, M.D., believes America has a public social/health crisis on its hands, and the doctor is fired up to do something about it.

Although outspoken and passionate, she is dedicated to her mission and advocates prevention and public health education as ways to make Americans healthy people. In her way of thinking, Americans have a prime opportunity to take a long, hard, critical look at where we are in our present health care situation. She also sheds much light concerning where it is we need to be if 'indeed' we even hope to achieve the goal of a healthy American people.

"The health of our nation is inextricably tied to the health of our citizens," she says. *"in order to meet the challenges of the Twenty-first Century, we must have a healthy America. We must have citizens who are capable of leading socially and economically productive lives; right now we don't have that. We have smoked up, drunk up, eaten up, messed up and used up our precious bodies far too long. It is time to do something about it."*

There are numerous ways to view what the doctor says. One way is to refrain from dividing ourselves by applying liberal and conservative labels to ourselves. Maybe we could help each other to see ourselves as "learners" with

Joycelyn Elders as a doctor/teacher. What real conclusions can be drawn from what she prescribes?

There is a cartoon which pictures a patient wearing a hospital gown which exposes his rear end. The caption reads, "Health Care: You only think you're covered." Dr. Elders believes that many of us under our present health care system have our rears exposed.

Is she on target and timely in her assessment of the situation? Is the present arrangement producing a healthy America? Are we trashing our most valuable resource, our children? Honestly, aren't there many problems and inequities in the delivery of healthy care today based on race, sex age and economics? Are we confusing the issues of morality and public health?

For simply stating her views (which have been misrepresented) and trying to provoke thought, she has been attacked again and again for her stands on sex education, contraception, and teenage pregnancy; she has received criticism for proposing alternatives to spending tens of billions of dollars each year on national drug policy that so far seem more effective at filling prisons and convicting first-time offenders than preventing and curing drug addiction and the spread of AIDS. Some congressmen even called for her resignation because she suggested the possibility of studying the chance of researching the legalization of drugs as an alternative to current United States drug policy.

For her progressive positions on the issues, the doctor is on fire, under fire and fired! She has been tried, but the jury is still out in the former Surgeon General's case.

We may not learn the real verdict in her case until sometime in the next century. We should not be surprised if she is found "not guilty" of the unclear charges against her, charges made by embarrassed Democrats who were delivered a major defeat by the Republican Party in the November, 1994 election. For their loss the Democratic Party's leadership made the first African-American U.S. Surgeon General the first scapegoat. A quick trial was held in her absence: the prosecuting attorney was Leon Panetta, the jury was Donna Shelala, and the sentencing was carried out by the judge/best friend who fired her. Is the case closed? Only the American people can answer that question.

The conservative tide sweeping America today seems to be made up of people who are unable to see beyond the status quo, people who take a selfish and narrow view of things. Anyone who rocks their boat is destined for dismissal of one kind or another. Unabashed by the reality of this situation in America, Joycelyn Elders did not stop speaking, she did not sit down, she did not turn back because she found it too hard; she kept on "dancing with the bear."

The lesson being taught us with regard to our health care system is that we do not have time to continue fighting among ourselves, moralizing, demoralizing, etc. There is work to be done, and Dr. Elders is trying to teach us the new attitude that this work requires. She is saying that we need to reorder our priorities and our thinking. If we think that we can continue to live as we are and be successful in health care, we are already dead. The failures of the present way should make us realize our mortality. We know, of course, that as human beings our mortality is a given, but what troubles Dr. Elders is that we seem so bent on hastening the process!

It may be that those who make up "the bear" have criticized and attacked Dr. Elders, the "lightning rod," for her stand because they would like to maintain the status quo that benefits only them. You see, "the bear" is usually the comfortable middle-class who shroud their children in the best of schools, the best insurance policies, and the most select cultural and social activities, and whose churches segregate themselves on Sunday morning for worship. Yet these are the people who seem to think they have some inalienable right to engage in moralizing and determining what is best for our children, women's reproductive rights, etc.

Dr. Elders understands that to reach the level of health care and education that she believes is right for this country, coalition-building must be a part of the plan. She wants "the bear" to join in and understand that the people deserve better than they are getting. She wants Americans to feel too that they have power over their situation. She bequeaths to us her convictions about health care. Until we can come together on the issues, M. Joycelyn Elders, M.D. says not to worry about her: she is still just as strong in her convictions as always; "though pressure may be brought to bear, despite the consequences, she stands firmly there," still Dancing with the Bear.

WORKS CITED

Anonymous. Complete Speakers and Toastmasters Library. Ed. Jacob M. Braude. Englewood Cliffs, NJ: Prentice Hall, 1965.

Atkins, Norman. "Respect Your Elders." Family Life July-August 1994:62+.

The Bible. Quotations from: King James Version, New English Bible, New International Version, New Revised Standard Version, Revised Standard Version.

Blount, Carolyne S. "A Caring Crusader." About...Time April 1991:13+.

"Can You Rely on Condoms?" Consumer Reports March 1989: Cover, 135+.

Children 1990. Children's Defense Fund. Washington: Children's Defense Fund, 1990.

Elders, M. Joycelyn. "America's Children: Our Vision of the Future" National Coalition of Equality in Learning, 24 Jan. 1992.

— — "Children, Poverty and Health"

— — and Jennifer Hui. "Comprehensive School Health Services: Does It Matter and Is It Worth the Fight?" Council of Chief State School Officers, Summer, 1992.

— — "'Conflict Goes with the Territory'" Editorial USA Today 12 Dec. 1994: 12A.

— — "Portrait of Inequality." Meharry Medical College "Targeting Needs of the Underserved: The Urgency of Health Care Reform" 5-6 Oct. 1992.

– – "The Renaissance of Empowerment." National Black Methodists for Church Renewal 27th Annual Meeting 26 Mar. 1994.

– – "Student Health Crisis: A Response for School Administrators." National Chief State Educators Fall, 1992.

– – Sonoma County Physician Foreword, Manuscript: Final Version.

– – "Talk Alive" CNBC. April, 1993.

Fullerton, Jane. "Elders Goes Under Senate Knives Today." Arkansas Democrat Gazette 23 July 1993, sec. A:1+.

Graham, Judith, ed. Current Biography Yearbook. New York: W. Wilson, 1992.

Green, Ernest J. Personal Relationship, An Approach to Marriage and Family. Boston: McGraw Hill, 1978.

Haselden, Kyle. The Racial Problem in Christian Perspective. New York: Harper Brothers, 1959.

Hilts, Philip J. "Blunt Style on Teen Sex and Health." New York Times 14 Sept. 1993, sec. C:1+.

Johnson, John H. Succeeding Against the Odds. Washington: Amistad Pr., 1993.

Lawson, J.M. Letter to President Clinton. 20 Dec. 1994. Used by permission.

Leveritt, Mara. "An Informant's Story." Arkansas Times 16 Dec. 1994: 13+.

Myrdal, Gunnar. An American Dilemma. New York: Harper Brothers, 1944.

Nimmons, David. "Playboy Interview: Joycelyn Elders." Playboy. June 1995: 55+.

Outler, Albert C. John Wesley. New York: Oxford University Press, 1964.

Phillips, Mary Christine. "Taken for Granted Again." Black Issues in Higher Education 19 Dec. 1994: 28+.

Pincus, Ward. "Elders' Son, 28, Pleads Innocent to Drug Charge." Arkansas Democrat Gazette 21 Dec. 1993, sec. B:1+.

Rowan, Carl T. Breaking Barriers. Boston: Little, Brown, 1991.

Russell, Greg. "Ready for Battle." UAMS Journal. Summer, 1993: 24+.

Schwartz, John. "Elders Faces Confirmation Hearing Today." The Washington Post 23 July 1993, sec. A:4.

– –"Hearings on Surgeon General Nominee Postponed." The Washington Post 16 July 1993: 1+.

Sine, Tom. Wild Hope: Living with Confidence in the Face of Future Shock. Dallas: Word, 1991.

Stumpe, Joe. "Elders' Talk Spotlights LR House." Arkansas Democrat Gazette 11 Dec. 1993, sec. A:1+.

United States Cong. Joint Committee on Printing. Congressional Record. 103rd Cong., 1st sess. Washington: GPO, 7 Sept. 1993.

United States Dept. of Health & Human Services. Public Health Service Commissioned Corps. Washington: GPO.

United States Gov't Printing Office. <u>Hearing of the Committee on Labor and Human Resources United States Senate</u>. 103rd Cong., 1st sess. Washington: GPO, 23 July 1993.

Voltaire, Francois-Marie A. de. "Candide." <u>The Norton Anthology of World Masterpieces.</u> Volume 2, 4th Edition Ed. Maynard Mack, et.al New York: Norton, 1979

Ward, Harry P. "Time in the Trenches." Editorial. <u>UAMS Journal</u>. Summer, 1993: 2.

INDEX

A

Affirmative Action 205
American Social Thought and History 217
Ansell, Inc. 122
Arkansas Area - The United Methodist Church i, vi
Arkansas Children's Hospital iv, 69, 212
Arkansas Department of Health iv, 4, 73, 103, 106, 108, 109, 118, 121, 134, 137, 145, 146, 152, 157, 171
Arkansas Health Department *See Arkansas Department of Health*
Arkansas Times 195
Asso. of State and Territorial Health Officers 145, 152

B

Berry, Mary Frances 217
Bethesda, Maryland 211
Black History Week 52
Black Issues in Higher Education 217
Boxer, Barbara 162, 163
Boyle Park 178, 189
Breaking Barriers 124, 156
Bridgeway Treatment Center 192
Brooklyn Dodgers 220
Brooks Army Medical Hospital 67, 68
Brown, Ron 221
Bumpers, Dale 106, 163
Bush Administration 224
Bush, George 224
Butler, Tom 121
Byrd, Mrs. 183, 184

C

Central High School 197, 198
Chicago, Illinois 18
Children 1990 - A Report Card, Briefing Book, and Action Primer 122
Christian Methodist Episcopal(CME) Church 80
Cisneros, Henry 221
City of Little Rock 178
Civil Rights 204, 205
Clark, Dr. 214, 215
Clinton Administration 214, 219
Clinton, Hillary Rodham 202
Clinton, William Jefferson "Bill" i, 4, 15, 51, 66, 95, 103, 109, 111, 120, 168, 171, 174, 181, 188, 197, 210, 211, 213-215; 221, 223, 224
Coats, Dan 113-115; 150, 158, 159
Cole, Johnnetta 219, 223
"Crossing the Bar" 52

D

Delta Sigma Theta Sorority 63
Denver, Colorado 67
Department of Health and Human Resources 113, 147
Department of Health and Human Services 109, 121, 191, 211

233

Detroit, Michigan 32
Dillard, Hattie 17, 18
Dillard, Tom 17, 18
Dillard, William 18, 38
Dillard's Department Stores 18, 198
Dillard's Dry Good Store 17
Donaldson, Charles ii
Dunbar, Paul Lawrence 52
Durenberger, Dave 159

E

Eisenhower. Dwight D. 197
Elberta Drive-In Theatre 207
Elders, Eric i, 6, 73, 100, 101, 180, 184 -186, 187
Elders, Grandmother 101
Elders, Kevin i, 6, 100, 178-181; 183- 188; 190-194; 196
Elders, Kevin Maurice 179, 180
Elders, M. Joycelyn i-vi; 1, 3 -14; 16 - 23; 25, 29- 35; 37-41; 43- 45; 48-52; 54-79; 86, 96, 99-101; 103-106; 108-122; 126, 128-130; 132- 140; 143-151; 156-1 66; 168-172; 174-179; 181, 183-1 85; 188-194; 197, 199, 202, 203, 205-208; 210-215; 217-223; 225, 226, 228
Elders, O.B. *See Elders, Oliver*
Elders, Oliver i, 6, 99-102; 112, 113, 115, 116, 118, 148, 167, 177, 178, 180, 181, 183, 185, 189, 192, 211, 212
Elders, Oliver B. *See Elders, Oliver*
Espy, Mike 221

F

Flight, Claude 102
Food and Drug Administration 121
Fort Bragg, N.C. 77
Fort Smith, Arkansas 6
Foster, Henry 95, 204, 221
Fox, Fanny 197
French, Marilyn 200
Frisk, Rev. 41

G

G.I. Bill 69, 77, 152
George Washington Bridge 179
Glenview Community 183, 185
Glenview Elementary School 185
Global Gathering Ministries 8
Grambling University 188
Gray, Sonya Hunt 191
Green, Ernest J. 213, 216
Guinier, Lani 219,223

H

Henry, Patrick 211
Herman, Alexis 148
Hicks, Kenneth 1
Hightower, Sgt. 208
Hill Brother's Place 15, 17
Holiman United Methodist Church 223
Holladay, Charles 179
Hollingsworth, P.A. "Les" 180
Hollingsworth, Perlesta A. 190
Hope, Arkansas 15
Horace Mann High School 99
Houston, Texas 63, 67
Howard County, Arkansas 1, 3, 4, 15, 80

Howard County Training
   School 51, 57
Howard University 6
Hunter United Methodist
   Church 192

I

Indianapolis, Indiana 8
Internal Revenue Service 180

J

J.B. Hunt Trucking Co. 198
J.D. 47
Jackson, Mississippi 208
"Jesus Loves Me" 86
Johns Island, S.C. 6
Johnson & Johnson Personal
   Products 188
Johnson, Lyndon 156, 205
Jones, Bernard
   i, 6, 19, 48, 61
Jones, Beryl 19, 62, 81
Jones, Charles 19, 48, 49, 61
Jones, Charlie 14, 15, 38, 57
Jones, Chester R. ii, 11, 19,
   62
Jones, Curtis 2, 14-16; 18-
   20; 22, 26-28;
   32, 34, 40-42; 47-50; 57-
   59, 62, 72, 73, 80,
   84, 88, 95
Jones, Edith Irby 3, 63, 77
Jones, Fred 59, 61
Jones, Haller 2, 12-16;
   18, 19, 22, 23, 26, 32-
   34; 41, 45, 48-50; 58,
   59, 61, 72- 74; 80 -82;
   84-86; 89-91; 93-95
Jones, Herbert, Jr. 188, 195
Jones, Katie
   19, 32, 40, 48, 61
Jones, Kevin 101
Jones, Little Minnie. *See*
   Elders, M. Joycelyn

Jones, Minnie
   14, 15, 29, 57, 63
Jones, Minnie Lee. *See* Elders,
   M. Joycelyn
Jones, Pat 6, 19, 62
Jones, Phil 19
Jones, Valarie A. i,
   210, 211
Jones, Will 19, 80

K

Kansas City, Kansas 76
Kansas City, Missouri 26, 64
Kassebaum, Nancy 54
Kennedy, Edward M. i, 117,
   119, 120, 149,
   150, 157, 158, 160,
   161, 165
King, Rodney 204
Kipling, Rudyard 52
Koop, C. Everett 167, 173,
   217, 218
Korean War 66, 67

L

Lake Pine Bluff 186
Lakewood Subdivision 185
Lambert, Blanche 157
Lawson, J.M., Jr. 223, 224
*Let Down Your Bucket Where
   You Are* 57
Lincoln, Abraham 32, 205
"Little Minnie". *See* Elders, M.
   Joycelyn
Little Rock, Arkansas 6, 58,
   59, 64, 99,
Little Rock Police Department
   178-
   180; 188, 189, 194, 195
Little Rock Public Library 52
Little Rock School District
   198, 199

Los Angeles, California 204, 223
Louisville, Kentucky 122

M

MacArthur Park 66
MacArthur, Douglas 66
Mandela, Nelson i
Marcia Cove 185
McCain Shopping Mall 185
McCracken, Branch 102
Meredith, James 208
Metzenbaum, Howard M. 158
Mills, Wilber 197
Milwaukee, Wisconsin 66, 67
Mine Creek 15
Mineral Springs, Arkansas 17, 18, 67, 80
Mormon Tabernacle Choir 41
Morton, Eva Moore 64
Moseley-Braun, Carol 161, 220, 221
Mother Sabie 2, 16, 19
Myrdal, Gunnar 204

N

NAFTA 224
Nashville, Arkansas 59, 207
National Bank of Arkansas 112, 114, 115
National Geographic Society 6
National Health Core 211
National Institutes of Health iv, 152
National Organization of Women 200
National Press Club 177, 179
New York, N.Y. 214
Nickles, Don 113-115; 129, 132, 148
Nimmons, David 171
Nina 6, 100, 101

Norplant 129, 133
North Little Rock, Arkansas 183, 185, 188
North Little Rock Bank Board 114
Novello, Antonia C. 167

O

"Old Yeller" 51, 207, 208, 218
Ole Miss. *See* University of Mississippi
O'Leary, Hazel 219
Oxford, Mississippi 208
Ozan, Arkansas 14

P

Palmer, Chris 195
Panetta, Leon 223, 227
Park Plaza Mall 210
Personal Relationships, An Approach to Marriage and Family 213, 216
Philadelphia, Pennsylvania 191
Philander Smith College 3, 58-61; 63, 64, 66, 74, 118, 151, 187, 207
Phillips, Mary Christine 217
Pine Bluff, Arkansas 179
Playboy 171
Plegge, John 189, 190
President's Council on Physical Fitness and Sports 167
Public Health Service 151, 152, 157, 167, 168
Pulaski County Circuit Court 189
Pyramid Club 63

R

Reed, Charlie 14, 18
Reed, Elnora 14, 18, 48

Reed, Jeff 18, 19
Reid, Beryl 49
Reid, Charlie 49
Reynolds, Cornelius 66, 68
Richmond, California 49- 51; 53
Robinson, Jackie 220, 221
Rogers, Doyle 28
Rogers, Raye 28
Roman Catholic Church 145
Roosevelt, Fanklin 165
Rowan, Carl T. 124, 156

S

Saline River 15
Schaal, Arkansas 1, 2, 15, 18, 34, 48, 50, 58, 80, 83, 118
Schwartz, John 167
Scott, J.D. 61, 62, 63
Segal, Geraldine R. 217
Senate Committee on Labor and Human Resources 113, 116, 147
Sewell, Joella 26, 64
Shalala, Donna 109, 227
Sine, Tom 139
Sonoma County Physician 170
Southern Baptist Convention 204
Spellman College 223
St. Paul, Minnesota 64
Stephens Family 198
Stephens, " Mr. Whitt" 197, 198

T

Tabernacle Christian Methodist Episcopal Church 32
Tabernacle CME Church 80, 83
"Taken for Granted Again" 217
"Talk Alive" 129
Talmadge, Herman 164
TCBY 198
Teel, Gina ii
Terry, Luther 173
"The 5-H Club" 9, 144, 15
The Arkansas Democrat-Gazette 178, 179
The Arkansas Times 190
The Farmer's Almanac 39
The Washington Post 167
Tollette, Arkansas 57
Tom, Dr. 64
Truman, Harry S. 66, 163
Tucker, Jim Guy 197
Tunk 47
"Tweet" 195
Tyson Foods 198

U

U.S. Army 3, 5, 66, 76, 77, 118, 152, 208
U.S. Army 82 Airborne Division 77, 208
U.S. Constitution 218
U.S. Department of Education 211
U.S. House of Representatives 177
U.S. Supreme Court 219, 220
U.S. Surgeon General iv, 1, 5, 8, 10, 17, 34, 44, 54, 74, 88, 106, 112-114; 116, 119, 120, 124, 129, 138, 143, 145, 158-162; 166-168; 170-173; 175, 177, 179, 188, 189, 192, 193, 203, 204, 210-212; 217, 218, 220, 225-227
UAMS College of Medicine See University of Arkan-

sas College for Medical Sciences
Uncle Bud 81
United Nations 211
United Methodist Church 7, 8, 151. *Also See Arkansas Area-United Methodist Church*
United Nations 214
United Press International 179
United States Public Health Service 173
University of Arkansas at Fayetteville 187
University of Arkansas at Little Rock ii
University of Arkansas College of Medicine's Endocrine Division 70
University of Arkansas Medical Center 69
University of Arkansas School for Medical Sciences iv, 3, 4, 63, 69, 99, 152, 212
University of Indiana 102
University of Minnesota iv, 3
University of Minnesota School of Medicine 69
University of Mississippi 208
University of Pennsylvania 217
USA Today 172

V

Virginia State College i
Virginia State University 102

W

WAC 66, 67
Wal-Mart Corporation 28, 197, 198
Walker, General 208
Wallis & Wallis Advertising ii
Wallis, Dave & Ernie ii